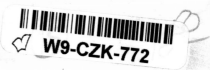

LOCKED

INTO

LIFE

LOCKED IN TO LIFE

Patton Howell *and* James Hall

Tea Road Press

P.O. Box 16590
Boise, Idaho 83715
www.tearoadpress.com

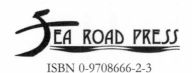

ISBN 0-9708666-2-3

Printed in the United States of America

Library of Congress Cataloging-in-Publication Data

Howell, Patton, 1921-
Locked in to life / by Patton Howell and James Hall.
p. cm.
Includes index.
ISBN 0-9708666-2-3 (Hardcover)
1. Hall, James, 1934---Health. 2. Cerebrovascular
disease--Patients--Texas--Biography. 3.
Psychiatrists--Texas--Biography. I. Hall, James, 1934- II. Title.
RC388.5.H35 H69 2002
362.1'9681'0092--dc21
2002007372

Acknowledgements

We, James Hall and Patton Howell, want to thank our editors, Megan Howell and Marcelline Watson, for making this book possible. Our deep and lasting appreciation to you both.

Our wives suffered with us through the writing and contributed substantially. We owe you a sincere debt of gratitude and also the colleagues who took time from their overloaded schedule to read the manuscript.

Special thanks to our publisher Rhonda Winchell Sharp, who wonderfully loved the book and has made many loving suggestions for making it better.

Table of Contents

Resources

Index

I

Stroke

Mind

The separation of mind from body is one of human kinds oldest and most persistent beliefs. Skulls from ancient burial sites sometimes have little round holes drilled in the tops. These little holes are a message of fear sent across the millennia. The holes are a way to get out. They were inspired by the fear of one's mind existing forever locked up in a useless dead body. That is how the idea of ghosts may have originated. It was also a primitive concept of soul.

Today the meaning of soul can be found in a special kind of stroke called the Locked-in Syndrome. Think of the grisly meaning of "locked-in." It means that the mind of a person who suffered this kind of stroke is locked into a body to which it has lost all connection. The body seems dead. Are these people lying motionless in their hospital beds still human? Do they have conscious minds trapped in their bodies? It is possible that the minds of some of the victims of Locked-in Syndrome are kicking and fighting to get out of those coffin-like bodies, seeking those little holes that our ancestors drilled into the skulls of their dead.

Losing touch with one's body and still being a locked-in mind is one of humanity's basic fears. How much of a mind can one have without a body? Without contact with the body does the mind drift off into a grey kind of nothingness? When there are no senses, feelings, or stimuli from the body, how can the self exist? Would one go mad from mentally beating against the sides of a coffin-body? There are nightmares like this. Folk tales and B movies are littered with such horrors.

Stroke is not an illness. There is no single infection or disability to "cure." Cells of the brain have died. They will not come back to life. Each case of stroke is unique in itself and is related to the development of a person's whole life. Stroke survival is a metamorphosis, a rebirth of brain function. What can mind do when it has no body? It can think rather than act. This is a breakthrough in understanding what it means to be a human being.

Will we be locked in to death or locked in to life? The answer is in the story of a man, Dr. James Hall, who chose life. He was a victim of the Locked-in Syndrome. The metamorphosis of his brain being reborn will lead him into a new spiritual existence. He tells how living as a mind extends toward eternity. Beyond, there is something beautiful.

Judgement Day

Thursday morning, April 11, 1991. Dr. James Hall woke early, and looking through his closet, picked a designer Harris tweed suit, white shirt, coordinated tie. A light topcoat. No, not the one cut like an opera cape. This trip was to Akron. Here, this London Fog trench coat would be appropriate. He didn't wake his wife Susy to say goodbye. In fact, he hardly noticed her.

Leaving his rambling ranch style house in fashionable North Dallas, he drove his Jaguar sports car to his psychiatric office. There he returned a call from the manager of his ranch in West Texas, saying he would be out there in a few days to oversee the year's branding of cattle. Later in the day he was on the Lyndon Baines Johnson Freeway to the complex sprawl of roads and terminals that is the Dallas/Ft. Worth International Airport. He got to the airport and found the flight to Akron delayed.

Then there was a second delay. It was late in the day when he finally settled back comfortably in his first class seat. The stewardess brought him a few drinks and spent the rest of the flight coming on to him.

During the flight he sensed that something was wrong. He just made it to the men's room and vomited. He almost never vomited. Maybe he had had too much alcohol.

Getting the rental car was a chore as usual. The gearshift on the rental car seemed awkward; he felt disoriented. He felt a fretful need for his own sports car. This was not his Jag. Something felt urgent. What is....Hospital! Had to find a hospital. It was hard to read the signs....a half an hour went by....where was he? Lost. He was lost to begin with. A truck stop loomed ahead. He parked the rental car somehow and dashed through the rain. It was late at night and there were few customers around. The restaurant was closed except for one section. He needed to urinate badly. Where were the restrooms? He spotted the women's room first. The men's room usually adjoins it. It did! He urinated just in time. Now he must ask for directions. He looked at their candy. Should he buy something since he used their facilities? Forget it – it was probably not the first time it had happened. He approached the girl behind the counter. She seemed frightened. Did he look as if he were going to rob her?

"I am just lost." He tried to explain, and words became a jumble.

She looked at him in alarm. He couldn't even understand himself and stumbled off. The rain had become a slow drizzle as he fumbled to unlock the rental car. He drove off into the strange black night, on and on.

Suddenly there was a loud ringing in his ears. He spotted a graveled shoulder at the edge of the road. He pulled over, put the car in neutral, and leaned his head back on the car seat. The ringing didn't go away. Ahead through the slow rain he saw what looked like an official building of some kind. Behind it there were parking spaces. The ringing got louder, and he put the car into drive and watched for an opening in the traffic. One comes and he eases the car across the highway, stops in front of the building. LEGS. THE LEGS. HEAD PAIN. PAIN. PAIN. PAIN. His head was full of sharp knives cutting and tearing his brain. He turned off the motor. His body fell onto the horn. Its sound seemed lost in the night. The rain fell only occasionally now.

After a long time, a man opened the back door of the building and came to the car window, holding a raincoat draped over his head.

"Can I help you?"

James' head in the car couldn't move. After receiving no response the man went away. Soon a kind ambulance attendant arrived. "Are you all right?" he asked gently.

No answer, just the blaring horn of the rental car. The attendants got him out of the car and strapped onto a stretcher. They took his suitcase into the ambulance. He couldn't speak. He worried about the billfold in his pocket.

Upside down traffic lights. Ambulance. The wheels of the metal stretcher click, click, click. He couldn't see but knew the smells and noises of a hospital. Emergency room blur. Screened off cubicle. In a surge towards life, he seemed to be sitting up, saying something. An intern came in and took his blood pressure. The intern hurried to the phone. CONVULSIONS. He felt his body slipping away. So this was the way death came ....Consciousness was obliterated in a final stabbing pain in his head.

When the intern returned, he found a still, cold body lying on the table. There was no response.

Locked-in

Susy, James' wife, told me how she had groggily answered the phone at five the next morning. The Akron hospital told her that Dr. Hall was there with a serious, life and death, stroke. Susy flew to Akron. At the hospital she was greeted by a visibly embarrassed doctor who told her that another woman was already there to take care of James. Susy said, "Then in that case she can have him." Later, overwhelmed with grief and pain, she said she had found herself waiting in the doctor's office. He came in and told her that the woman had left the hospital. She was not coming back. Susy stayed. One of James Hall's patients provided a private airplane to fly his body home from Akron to Dallas.

James had dominated Susy all their lives. Now she was the one in charge. In Dallas she called me, Patton Howell, a forensic psychophysiologist (mind/brain interface), for help. I will be telling the story of his stroke.

I came down the hall. The staff of the teaching hospital had assigned James a suite. I approached the door and leaned my head against it for a moment and tried to prepare myself for what lay within. Susy slipped out as I opened the door. She thanked me for releasing her and went off down the hall to do some errands.

It was like breaking into a sepulcher. The room was absolutely still. It had the atmosphere of an empty room, as if no one were alive there. The featureless walls and ceiling blurred into a chaos without form or sensation. I approached the bed slowly and contemplated James' body. James had been going bald for years. Now there were just a few graying hairs scattered over his massive round head. His skin was cold. It had no resilience. His whole body was absolutely still, like a laid-out corpse.

Think of someone's face. Even in sleep there are subtle signs of awareness of the outside world, imperceptible movements around the eyes and mouth. The skin has a radiance of life that reaches out and touches you. When a person is dead, that radiance disappears. The tone of life is gone.

I reached over and pushed the skin of James' face. Nothing. I pushed the flesh of his shoulder. It was like pushing a shoulder of beef at the grocers, no response, no tingle of life. Suddenly my hand darted out to the carotid artery in James' neck. Yes, his body was alive.

I realized I had been holding my breath. I collapsed into a chair by the bed and tried to read, for the second time, the data on James that I had brought from the MRI laboratory.

Problems of brain and mind were my field and one in which I had written extensively. In a moment I gave up, my face sinking into my hands. Suddenly I stood up, went over to the basin to wash my face. After carefully drying it, I began pacing across the room, waiting for Bill Moore, a friend and colleague of James. I had asked him to meet me today.

It was a nice room with an alcove off the side with a couch and table and three chairs. There was a comfortable easy chair in the room with James. The furniture was clean, but institutionalized brown. My depression at James' reported condition was intensified by the room. The walls were white, the ceiling white, the doors white. No pictures on the walls, not even in the alcove. It was superior for a hospital, all the necessary fixtures to keep the body alive. All those who work around hospitals get used to the smells of sickness, but suddenly I was very aware of it. The structure of the building emanated it. It expressed a fear and horror held in from the outside world. All this flashed through my mind in an instant.

Bill, bearded, muscular, came in. He always looked as though he would be more comfortable outdoors. He had overseen the training of two generations of psychiatrists at the Southwestern Medical School here. Bill was known to be a mountain of strength in crises such as this, but now he appeared pale and haggard. The reports of his old friend's condition left his eyes brimming in pain.

We two held each other for a moment by the bed, and then Bill slid into a chair and I began to pace. It was time for action. These were critical moments. As far as I could tell the only brain scan that was done was Magnetic Resonance Imaging. That was OK, but it only told which brain cells were still alive. I wished we had Positron Emission Tomography on this. It would tell us if any brain cells were being used – for thinking, for example.

I had guessed that James' body was permanently gone. This was the classic Locked-in Syndrome. The statistical chance for survival was one out of ten. More than that, what was the chance of a meaningful life without his body? The statistics on this hardly gave James a chance.

Bill was standing by the bed contemplating the still figure. There wasn't any thinking going on. I knew how hard it is to get Positron Emission Tomography set up. And in a critical situation like this we would all just concentrate on what was vital first. The facial muscles had no tone at all.

I moved to Bill's side, James' face emphasized his corpse-like appearance. That was what had been frightening me.

The lack of tone implied that the stroke must have occurred in the pons area.

I showed Bill the sketch I made in the lab. An artery split in the mid-brain by the pons. Apparently there was a blockage, probably cholesterol, in the artery which caused the split. Not only did brain cells die from lack of blood supply but they were traumatized by the pressure of blood leaking from the split artery. I guessed that this mid-brain pons area had been wiped out with much of the lower cortex including the thalamus and hyperthalamus traumatized by the flood of blood. We had a Locked-in Syndrome.

Bill sat down staring off into space. Then he turned to me and asked if I remembered that experiment with decorticated cats. I asked him to describe it. He told how the cat's cortex was removed by cutting through the nerves and separating it from the lower-brain, which remained functioning. Removing the cat's cortex guaranteed that there would be no neural impulses from its higher brain. The decorticated cat's body would just lie there living, but immobile unless stimulated. Then you put a decorticated cat in a cage with other cats, they don't react to its presence. Even when you stimulated the decorticated cat to an unconscious rage – snarling, fangs exposed, claws extended, the other cats ignored it. It was as though they thought of it as dead.

Bill's point was that others, even including overworked doctors and nurses, might have similar reactions to James. We would have a new syndrome – The Decorticated Cat Syndrome.

Bill, as usual, had struck to the point of James' life right now. If he had any mind left, it would need a positive environment. Magnetic Resonance Imaging showed that some brain cells in James' cortex were still alive. Unlike the decorticated cats, James still has his cortex in place even though it was disconnected from his body.

I remembered a Locked-in Syndrome case – as I recalled they had used Magnetic Resonance Imaging there without Positron Emission Tomography – the same situation we had here with James. The neurosurgical team there said that unfortunately, prolonged survival was possible. Notice the word "unfortunately." It was the Decorticated Cat Syndrome in action.

Doctors here talked about the "awesome" nature of the patient's inability to move or communicate and how the family and hospital staff began to feel hopeless and incapacitated in the presence of the Locked-in Syndrome.

Then as Bill and I talked, we too slipped into the same behavior. We were talking beside James' apparently dead body instead of trying to communicate with him. Where were our emotions of grief and pain? They were inside us, but we couldn't be ruled by emotions when trying to save a life. Could we? I take a moment to go deeper even though this is a crisis. Bill and I were not emotionally dead. Love is an emotion and an energy that transforms us into action of the highest order.

Each of us came from very different backgrounds and points of view. Bill Moore, in his sixties, was anti-religious and anti-spiritual, in contrast to James Hall. My focus was on brain waves and the mind/brain interface. Over the years, we three diverse men had bonded into an effective unified team. Now one of us lies mute, and helpless in a hospital bed with a very uncertain future.

Bill rubbed his hands over his face as though to keep emotion out of its tired lines. He suggested an assumption – infer that the cortex was being supplied with blood but the nerve cells connecting the cortex to the body were dead. If he could think, but couldn't communicate to us or anyone else, then what kind of life could he have? But assume first, that he could think and second, that there was some way that he could communicate. Then he could have some kind of life.

Standing by his bed, I looked down at his dear dead face and wondered. How could he be thinking with no input from his cortex to his body to tell him he's alive, things like breathing, heart beating, muscular feedback? Assume that he might be able to hear, and perhaps got some feedback from his eyes eventually.

Get inside his head and try to think like he's thinking – that is, if he's thinking.

Bill and I decided that the first thing he would know or believe was that if he didn't keep thinking, his mind would unravel and disappear – he would cease to exist. The body thinking that had always been going on behind his conscious thinking would be gone. That was the thinking that had opened doors, that had watched where he was going, that had moved the goblet of Courvoisier to his lips. Now that was gone. He might be conscious that it had been there. But that place was now empty. When he couldn't think of any new thoughts, he would have to repeat old thoughts. He would have to keep repeating them over and over again. He would be propelled by the same reflex as someone holding on with all of his might to the edge of a chasm. If he let go, he would fall.

His body used to experience physical fear, such as the fear of falling – adrenaline pumping through the blood, muscles spasaming. But that was gone, with his body, no emotions. Still he would feel fear, yet it would be a different type, a disembodied fear of his mind fading away. It would be a subjective creation. He would have to continuously create himself.

Maybe he would be thinking, that what would he do without a body, without legs and arms, without a throat to speak, how would he stand to not be able to eat or drink, he who had lived for the lusts of the flesh?

In his life he had blatantly betrayed his wife with other

26

women, yet he would know without question that he could not lose her now or he would disintegrate. His thoughts might be how he will keep her with him wherever he is going, even into this nothingness.

As a scientist he had explored near-death experiences with great interest. His whole professional life had been dedicated to the observation of phenomena beyond the senses. For him, psychotherapy had been the art of absorbing other people's mental states. So he was used to thinking beyond his senses. That might help him now.

So that was our plan, Bill and I would first, try to protect him from the caregivers who might turn against him in the Decorticated Cat Syndrome – second, to learn to think like James, to share his own thoughts with him even though he could not communicate them.

Without a Body

The next day I was alone in James' room determined to talk to him as though he were really thinking. "James, let's try this. Are you aware of yourself – whatever you are – as a consciousness without a body? Do you have thoughts, but no bodily sensations? Do you feel as if you are drifting in a place with no light? It isn't dark, maybe, but it isn't light. There are simply no sensations. All you know for certain is that you are thinking. Do you hold on to thoughts like a drowning man holds on to a life preserver? Are you afraid to let go?" I asked him.

"Death! James, do you remember its odor staining the air, and your nose wrinkling in disgust? It seems as though you and I had often felt the urge to throw up in the presence of putrefying flesh, and eject that threat of mortality from our beings. Flesh we knew would be lost into the ground without a memory of its being. The way we still embalm flesh and put it into coffins – anything to avoid thinking of that irrevocable physical loss of flesh. Why am I thinking about rotting flesh? Of course! You don't know if you have a body, or if it is rotting. James, your body is alive, you just can't feel it."

Suddenly I thought, does James know he has a name? "You are James A. Hall, M.D.!" I hadn't thought about his name earlier. Mental survival had seemed more important. He is now a different kind of being. His mind is separated from his body. Yet in a strange kind of mental existence his essential self can still think in words that have physical origins even though his physical body is lost to him. After his physical body has gone, how can words still exist in his mind?

Words are produced in the brain. But thoughts have hardwired your brain since you were a baby so you can produce words. So thoughts, to brain, to words. Words are then communicated through the physicality of beating the air with the tongue while using the bellows of the lungs or, by physically writing them on paper, typing them on a computer. Thoughts had been the womb of words. Can mind now exist without body in the same way that thoughts have grown to non-material interiority from material origins?

Now that Bill and I had decided to live in James' mind as best we could, I tried to imagine him in this situation. His eyes are the only things still alive, but they're just wandering around. Obviously, he's not controlling his eyes, but maybe he can hear. Is he afraid of losing his self or of fading away without ever being able to communicate? I can't imagine what that feels like.

I said, "I hope you can sense me, James. I can imagine you are struggling to keep yourself together. I believe in your existence more than I have before. Don't lose faith in yourself in this isolation. That cannot happen. I believe. I believe your mind is still alive. Alive! How confusing. This turns everything inside out. We have always assumed that body was vital to existence. James, you may be existing without awareness of body."

I thought to myself, this was a fine pretension but where would we go from here?

Murder

Bill and I came into the hospital room; my flesh shivered. It seemed too cold so I turned the thermostat up.

The news of James' stroke had been spreading. Susy was kept busy answering the phone and explaining. She didn't have the stamina to keep it up. Also, visitors were beginning to fill up the room, talking over James' body. They were patients, colleagues and friends. Bill and I talked to everyone to keep as much pressure off Susy as we could.

An earnest tall thin man who was an internist commented, "Yes, I understand that James had agreed with our group that too many patients who have become vegetables are being artificially supported by advanced medical techniques."

A breathless young man added, "I've got the wording of the Euthanasia Ballot in Washington State right here. It says, 'Shall adult patients who are in a medically terminal condition be permitted to request and receive aid in dying from a physician?' That seems very safe and sensible, doesn't it?"

There was clearly a lot of unexpressed anger at James for leaving the people who had depended on him the most. Decorticated Cat Syndrome.

Bill pulled me aside and said, "They don't look at him. They look at each other over him. They talk loudly as though to deny James' presence. They would obviously be relieved if he would die. What effect does it have on James' mind – if it's still here? This is not a good situation for James. If he doesn't get worse by himself, he will be allowed to get worse. The pressure is building for his body to die. How can we resist it? Of course no one can even imagine that James might be thinking himself."

Their talking continued.

It was infuriating to me. As though talking just to Bill, I raised my voice, "Do people think they can trust physicians with their lives? Can a doctor predict how long a patient is going to live? Of course not. We're wrong all the time. No one can say whether you're 'terminally' ill. Doctors can predict on the average fairly well, but that doesn't tell people anything about how long they personally will live."

Several doctors responded at once. The conversations were flying above James' bed as though he was not there. It was beginning to resemble a wake. I said to Susy, "If James had some mental functions at this point, he would be infuriated. I bet he would be cussing them out. Chronic, unmitigated pain is the usual impetus for euthanasia. Whatever else James might be feeling, it isn't pain."

Bill responds, "Right on, Pat. Physicians are supposed to live by the idea that at least we will try to do no harm. The whole practice of euthanasia is anti-life. Physicians will start saying they're caring about life while they are deliberately killing it. I'm here to tell you, there's more to life than we know."

Still pretending I was just talking to Bill, "Do you know that the Netherlands have had a law similar to this Washington proposition for the last twenty years? Doctors in the Hague say that physicians have gotten so used to killing people that it has now become common to kill without consent. The doctors just certify them as deaths from natural causes. We have to look at the ethical aspects of killing people no matter what the compassionate reasons may be. Killing people has to fit in with our whole approach to living. If you start removing the ethical parts of the professional structure, it will fail. You will be left with indiscriminate killing. Remember that the holocaust started with Nazi doctors supporting mercy killings of dysfunctional people."

Even Bill, always in control, was losing it with the atmosphere in the room. He also spoke up, "I know that we have all been fighting to get the best care for crack babies regardless of the cost. Would we then kill a man like James who may still have one of the best minds available? Is it too expensive or burdensome to care for a man who has helped so many people?"

A small, chubby and pink-cheeked man, Dr. Herrer, pursed his lips judiciously, "I'm afraid it is often difficult to bear. Those are tragic cases, but they are complex. We have to be very careful with the facts. We have here, one might say, an organism with its head cut off. Thought processes depend on interactions with the whole body. Mind is simply another word for brain. If there are no brain interactions with the body there is no mind. That aspect is very simple."

I replied, "Are you familiar with the literature on brain waves? It shows that most brain cells spend their time in routine housekeeping activities, just keeping the body functioning. Our thoughts actually use a negligible percent of our brain cells. Mental patterns use our brains not the other way around."

Dr. Herrer cut in his face red, "I beg your pardon, I treat many people who are in better mental condition than Dr. Hall. They have more to live for than he does, and let me tell you that most of them die. My sixty hour week doesn't have time for intellectualism."

An elderly gray-haired woman psychiatrist supported Dr. Herrer. "Enough of this dithering. I know that James left a request that he be helped out of life if anything happened that would compromise his ability to function effectively. So that's the end of the matter. He would want it. His family should want it. Do it!"

The chic young woman who is a "special" friend of James said, "When someone needs to die and doesn't, it's such a burden on family and friends. When you think he might stay alive in this condition indefinitely, its just too much to bear. As an internist specializing in these cases, wouldn't you agree Dr. Herrer?"

Dr. Herrer nodded, turned and left the room.

Susy tugged at Patton's arm. "Everyone heard you. Was that nice?"

"No it wasn't nice, Susy. Why do I feel so good about it?"

A nurse came into the room and asked us to leave.

Susy was still standing in front of me, her candid brown eyes looking into mine. I said, "I'm sorry Susy. I guess I'm just making things harder for you. If only there were some way I could communicate with James. I'm trying to be where he is. Only I don't know where he is. What if he still exists — somewhere?"

The Underworld

Next day I was pacing beside the bed. I told James, "I'm trying to imagine your mind without a body. I'm imagining a red Russian round-bottomed doll just like your body, and you're telling dirty jokes as usual."

I leaned over, "Hey, James, wait a minute, this red doll I'm imagining as your disembodied self just told me a disgusting joke about shining a flashlight into a blonde's ear to make her eyes sparkle. Mm, is that funny? No. I don't know how to make it funny like you used to do. Anyway I'm trying to be in your mind, but I don't remember the jokes you used to tell."

I continued, "The exciting thing is, however, that I imagined the joke right after I tried to stimulate your mind. We may not be communicating verbally, but I'm trying to influence your mind by thinking like you. How is that possible? I believe it is. I believe that my thinking that joke was mutual communication."

That night I dreamed of James as a nest of red round-bottomed dolls. The largest was the James the world knew, then the James Susy knew, then the James Bill knew, then the James I knew.

Back at the hospital I addressed James, "We know your mind is still here even though you've lost your body. Is there any way you can get a second chance? Maybe you won't like it down here in Death's house. We have washed up on some strange shores in our mental adventures together, haven't we? I've got to get through to you! Just like in the myths of the underworld, you can't look back. You must look forward. But I must, I must go back in your life."

I added, "James, this is my professional position. Listen up. We have to understand your entire life to understand your stroke. Your stroke is not an illness. There is no single infection or disability to 'cure.' Cells of the brain have died. They will not come back to life. Each case of stroke is unique in itself and is related to the development of a person's whole life. Stroke survival is a metamorphosis, a rebirth of brain function. Your stroke is the unique story of your life. I'm going back to the beginning – to when I first knew you, maybe, we can figure out how we got to this time in this hospital room, to this death of brain cells."

Locked In To Life

II

The James That Patton Knew

Locked In To Life

Beginnings

I was in a small hotel auditorium, full of the haze of cigarette smoke. It was a time before smoking had become prohibited. At a Jungian Society meeting everyone smoked. I can still taste the nicotine in the air. The speaker was a compactly put-together psychiatric doctor, handsome with a leonine head, James Hall.

He was giving a speech, talking about evidences of mind as an immaterial force independent of brain and capable of reorganizing brain cells to express mental intent. He wound up the lecture with evidence of a single mental power influencing many people. His final statement was, "And in conclusion let me assure you that Freud's apocryphal statement that in dreaming of a cigar, the cigar is sometimes just a cigar, is erroneous. A Jungian would say that a mental cigar is never just a cigar."

After the applause, James sat down next to us. Bill Moore, also a psychiatrist, said "Why do you smell funny?" James replied, "Ah Bill, that is not a smell but a very expensive scent, a cologne whose name would mean nothing to you." Bill, James, and I, Patton, were colleagues.

As the meeting broke up, James met his wife, Susy. She was an appealing woman with a hesitant manner. She obviously adored her husband. James kissed her and suggested that she go on up to their hotel room, "I've got to meet with some people, and I'll be a little while."

Later I noticed James talking to an attractive young woman who had been introduced as applying for a position as a Jungian therapist. James was offering her a fine scotch liqueur, "fit for the gods." The woman giggled and moved close to him. Later I saw them enter an elevator together, his hand on her hip.

The Magician

Another meeting years later was at The Cipango Club, the exclusive haunt of the movers and shakers of Dallas. It lay at the edge of a two mile stretch of forested parkland. A clear stream ran over a bed of white limestone. The matching white walls of a nearby theater designed by Frank Lloyd Wright nestled among the green trees.

Within the club on the second floor, a private party was in progress, a celebration of the 50th birthday of Dr. James Hall. He had become one of the city's most successful and influential psychiatrists. I was once again in attendance. For his party, he was giving a magic show. He called up his daughter Angela and offered to saw her in half. Angela was an attractive golden-haired young woman in her twenties. She climbed willingly into the magic box, and her father closed her inside, head and feet protruding, and sawed her in half. Then he separated the two sections of the box to show that she had indeed been cut in half. Then he put the two sections back together, opened the box, and out popped his whole living daughter. She gazed at him adoringly. He was the magician of life and death. The surrounding audience of mink-clad women and Armani-suited men clapped enthusiastically. One woman leaned over to whisper to another, "He's so wonderful. I've been going to him for seventeen years."

James seemed to gather all the light to himself as he stood assured and powerful amidst the rising applause. In the shadow off to one side was his wife, Susy. She was standing next to me. I noticed she was losing her figure. Her large and luminous brown eyes took in the scene.

I wondered what she was thinking about.

Susy said to me, "There is nobody like him, never was. He is one of a kind. His magic and his skills."

I was already in Dallas when James opened his practice there. He was elevated into a society where people too rich and sophisticated for Susy found titillations in sexual dalliances. Watching from the side of the room at the Cipango Club as her husband performed his tricks in the spotlight, Susy seemed overwhelmed by the feelings and rhythms of her past, perhaps of never quite belonging, of being ignored in social and professional conversations as an inconsequential and unwanted figure.

Later at a large conference at which James was the featured speaker I was sitting with Susy. James twice singled her meager accomplishments out for public ridicule. The second time this occurred, one of the analysts in the audience stood up and called him to account for his conduct. James laughed it off and suggested that if the analyst wanted to talk about it, he could visit him at his consulting offices as a patient – that is if he could afford James' exorbitant fees.

James loved the meetings, the groups, the heady surge of omniscient power. He bought a statue of Henry VIII, the English king who had six wives. He told his wife, "Susy, everyone needs a hobby."

Sex

It was fifteen years now that James and Bill and I had held monthly meetings at each other's homes. We compared notes and attempted to solve professional problems. Ours was an odd friendship. Socially we met infrequently. Professionally we were world's apart. Bill, a psychiatrist, was not impressed by theory, but rather regarded therapy as an art of feeling tones. James, also a psychiatrist, was a leader of the Jungian Society in the United States, and a prolific writer of books on hypnotism and Jungian theory of dreams. I was a psychophysiologist known for my research on brain waves and thought.

The publication of my first book, *Embodied Mind*, started our meetings. Bill, having read the book, brought James and I together to talk about some of its implications. Then our meetings became formalized to meet every month. We each seemed to have some aspect of our work that informed the other's problems. We became fast friends and enjoyed the meshing of intellects. Under Bill's supervision we taped all our meetings and I became the keeper of the archives. This evening we were meeting at James' home. James lived in a suitably grand house. I arrived to find Bill there sitting by a comfortable fire. James was in the bar mixing drinks.

We settled down with the taste of McClelland's 25-year-old scotch in our mouths and the smell of old leather upholstery in our nostrils. The fire warmed our bodies. James looked vulnerable.

Huddling in his chair he said, "We have become such good friends without talking about our personal affairs. Recently mine seem to have come crashing around my ears. Accusations against me will soon be well known in my social circle and among my Jungian colleagues. But I don't believe either of you know anything about this. I must admit that I have been dropped by social friends and by my colleagues. In fact, and this means a lot to me, you two are the only ones I trust right now. I need to tell you about my life from birth on. I am not feeling guilty. That is not healthy, but I am wounded, and to get through this with you I am going to have to be formal in tone. I'm going to have to ask you to let me monopolize this evening. We've solved so many problems with patients at these meetings. Now I want you to consider me the patient. I guess I'd better start with the early years of my marriage."

I am not going to continue quoting James. The story is too personal and I think is better told by someone else – by me in this case.

Sexual experiences, until James married Susy at twenty-one, were either disastrous or unsatisfactory. He didn't feel ready to marry. He was too young. But it was either marry then or lose the girl he loved. He still loves her and, despite a rocky road, he is still married to her. As strange at it seems in retrospect, it was not until about age forty that he felt himself to be sexually adequate. The other aspect of sex that contributed to his difficulties with sex was his expecting too much of it.

After his psychiatric residency at Duke, they went to the Jungian Institute in Zurich, Switzerland. Zurich reminded Susy of home, stable folksy lives and quiet old streets. The river running through Zurich reminded her of the one at home, placid and contained with sedate swans upon it. She would tell how she remembered that in the winter in Zurich, the clear water seemed black against the white snow. They had two daughters, Sherry and Angela.

In the 1970's when highly intelligent and motivated women began to be intrigued by the mysticism inherent in Jungianism, he was a major gatekeeper to the profession of Jungian psychoanalysis. He had actually certified many of the leading women analysts in practice. His lifestyle had supplied him with every sensual desire – rich sex and rich food along with high cholesterol and high blood pressure. He worked continuously giving international lectures, writing and attending to clinical practice. But he never for a moment thought of payback time.

Good food and drink were important to him. He judged Italian restaurants by the quality of their Zabigione – whether or not it was freshly made using an Espresso machine (which he preferred) and whether it was made with Marsala wine or a substitute like Sherry. Japanese restaurants, which were then rare in Dallas, were ranked by the quality of their Sushi and whether the menu offered Chowan Mushi, fish-soup custard.

After Zurich, he developed a taste for Fondue and Racklette, often cooking them at home. He became a fair chef, especially of Japanese dishes. His Crepes Suzettes were famous, as well as homemade eggnog, and an East Texas favorite – thin Country Ham with thick black coffee gravy.

His patron saint, Carl Jung, was a womanizer. James was just as discriminating about women as he had been about food, having a constant string of extramarital involvements. Most were simply mutually enjoyable, but five or six became serious. A mean-spirited Freudian once remarked that Jungian theory was an elaborate justification for making love to patients. James felt that love and pleasure were the very stuff of living and of psychotherapy.

His daughter, Angela, and his psychiatric nurse were very close. They worked together in his suite of offices. It was no secret that the nurse had been his lover since he opened his practice. In fact Angela and the nurse seemed to delight in humiliating Susy when she came to the offices.

Susy and James had been together since she was thirteen and lived on his street in the little town of Gladewater, Texas, an old town planted on the red sandy soil which gave the nearby Red River its name. The quiet streets were shaded by soaring Post Oak trees. Here was where they became sweethearts. Susy was a sweet pretty slip of a girl living with her aunt, feeling vulnerable without parents. James was everything she needed. He had been practicing magic since his childhood. His mother thought of him as a young genius. He was a high school class president twice and eventually valedictorian, powerful and successful.

His father was a successful real estate developer and his mother a chic modern woman of her time. There is a picture of James and his mother in the hallway. She was looking down at her four-year-old son with a passionate intensity, and he was looking up at her with the same devotion. The two of them remain frozen forever there on the wall in their own exclusive universe. We had all noticed the picture and what it revealed.

James graduated from the University of Texas magnum cum laude and Phi Beta Kappa. Susy got her degree in education near home at the Texas Christian University. When James asked her to marry him, she said she could never be worthy of him, but said yes anyway. She was whirled away into the chaotic and stressful life of medical school. James learned medicine; she taught elementary school.

One dark night she pressed her body against him and whispered, "Take me home James. Take me home."

James couldn't take her home. After medical school there was the war. He was a handsome dashing officer in the psychiatric corps. Away from Susy, he lived a full and exciting sexual life.

One day he was in a motel room with a lover and was interrupted by her estranged husband, a Green Beret instructor in close combat techniques. He expected the worst, but she handled the situation masterfully. He left. He realized that it would be impossible for him to continue the relationship. Later she said "You checked out when my husband came, didn't you? You never want to see me again." Her intuition amazed him. He did not want to admit he had run away.

Besides sex, another activity James was learning was drinking. One Sunday morning he wanted a drink but there was no liquor in the house. He suddenly realized that he never had alcohol around. The very next day he bought fifty dollars worth of liquor and put it in his kitchen cabinet. He became a regular and heavy drinker. But he was not guilty. His psychiatric training had taught him that guilt was unhealthy.

At the medical meetings psychiatric nurses would flop down beside him after he had given his lecture and rub their breasts against him. The psychiatric nurse from his office began to attend functions with him. She would sit on one side of him, pressed against him, her mouth to his ear, while Susy sat on the other side.

Susy had developed odd swellings all over her body. James had them too. A doctor friend had prescribed massive doses of penicillin for both of them. He had told Susy it was just something going around. Finally the woman responsible told Susy it was gonorrhea, so that Susy could protect her children. It became a dismal routine of bathroom hygiene, food, utensils. However, it finally all settled down without physically tragic results.

He frequently lectured to stimulating groups on Jung and hypnosis or various aspects of spirituality. Most groups were in the USA, but the list included Canada, England and Switzerland. He went to interesting meetings – Jungian, hypnosis and otherwise. Every four years, when there was an International Jungian Congress, he attended. This took him to Zurich, London, Rome.

He had stopped taking Susy with him. She had felt wretched while at the meetings, but she didn't want not to go. She had pled with him, begged him. He wouldn't take her, coldly brushing her feelings aside. It became obvious to Susy that a new young woman, married this time, found it necessary to go on the same trips as he did. Susy settled down with their two children in their new house trying not to think about things. She became a collector of small objects, withdrawing from the life around her.

James got up, "That brings us to the present. I think we need a break before I get to my present problems."

The Picture on the Wall

We each mixed new drinks of scotch. I had a double. This was a terrible story. I was looking at the picture of James and his mother. Finally I said, "James I've been worried about you for a long time."

He cut in with some of his old spirit, "Remember I don't feel guilty. That's unhealthy."

However, as James resumed his story, it got worse. He said, "At the close of the 1980's I was invited to an international conference, and I decided to take Susy. We were going to make a tour of Europe before the conference. Tickets, passports, hotel reservations for two, all a delightful rush getting ready. Finally Susy was dressed, packed and ready to go."

I'm going to take over the story again.

What happened next I'm afraid was burned into her soul. James came home and asked to see her ticket. Putting it in his pocket, he told her he had decided at the last minute to take someone else. He had fallen in love with another woman, someone new. He was going to let another woman use her ticket, fill her reservations at those romantic hotels. She cried, threatened divorce and begged on her knees clutching at him as he pulled away. He left her face down on the floor. Of all the things he had done to her this was too much for her to bear. (And for him although he denied any guilt.) And he did it anyway. Her heart had broken, the pieces grinding away in her breast. As she lay there sobbing James left and closed the door behind him.

His new mistress and he were in Europe making the Grand Tour. They ran into a colleague and his wife in Madrid's central park. The conversation seemed a little strained. The colleague declined an invitation to lunch and he and his wife hurried off.

He realized that they knew that Susy was supposed to be coming with him. Didn't expect to see someone else. He thought what business is it of theirs? He thought he had been up front and clear with Susy. But had he really been "up front?" Maybe he had just gotten used to not paying attention to her.

He pushed the thought away. It was of no consequence to him that his colleague, carrying this information with him, was on his way to Paris where the important psychological convention was to be held.

James thought that as long as he was comfortable with himself, he did not have to be concerned with what others might say. One of his maxims for psychological health was to never feel guilty. Under the hot Spanish sun among the sparkling fountains and green foliage of the park he and his friend spent a delightful afternoon. She was different from other women in his life who wanted some of his power. She didn't need anything from him. The image of the photograph of him and his mother regarding each other came into mind. Why would her presence stimulate that? An important connection. Other women with whom he had been sexually intimate had been in that picture. Each one became his mother in that forever world where he was the high school magician and nothing had consequences. Unfortunately that world only existed in an old photograph hanging on his wall. His liaisons gave the women what they wanted, but what did he want? Had he become his own cuckold, his own dupe? This woman was not in that picture. She was separate from him – tantalizing.

Another thing James had not considered was that he had made a date to be with his old mistress during the conference. With Susy it would have been no problem. That kind of dalliance went on routinely. But with this new woman it was different.

As it turned out, he missed the conference. He couldn't bring her to the conference because of his old mistress who was present. He sent the new mistress home. He tried to appease the old mistress by being with her the day after the conference, but she had heard the gossip about this new woman in his life, and she was angry. The whole trip ended in confusion and discomfort.

Everything was unraveling.

When he returned home, Susy was seeing a lawyer about a divorce. That was absurd. He told Susy, that that would mean giving her half of everything he had. He couldn't accept that. It was his!

"It's the law," said the lawyer.

In addition three other women in his life got together and filed ethics complaints against him.

This is ridiculous, he thought. They couldn't do that. He hired a lawyer who told him that yes, they could and even more, it was possible that monetary damages might be involved. He fought hard. The legal fees were substantial. This couldn't be happening to him.

But it did happen. He was thrown out of the local Jungian Society which he had dominated for so long. James hadn't noticed that those highly intelligent and liberated women he had been certifying as Jungian therapists were now in control of the Jungian Society.

As we left he said, "Defending myself on so many fronts simultaneously was a tremendous drain, both emotionally and financially. I felt no guilt whatsoever – they were vindictive and petty, in my mind, and I had done nothing but give them what they wanted."

The meeting broke up late without time for discussion. I felt James indeed needed some counseling from his friends. The stress on him must be unimaginable. Something was liable to break.

Bill and I knew that James was going to Akron to give a lecture the day after our meeting at his house. The days following his Locked-in stroke were so horrendous that no discussion was possible. A year passed before James could tell us the story of that judgement day.

III

The James That James Knew

Locked In To Life

The Mind of James Hall

I was talking to Bill, "Well, I think we understand something of the history of James' stroke – both the physical and the mental pressures that contributed to it. Remember the time-honored practice of doing the H & P, the history and the physical information of patients which you read in the process of doing rounds. You know how the H & P can be an essay about the unique quality of life of the patient. Depending on the physician who writes it, it can mean nothing or it can be life giving. Remember Larry Dossey, the internist and author of so many books on healing? I have an image of him warming his stethoscope between his two hands as though in prayer. He was getting prepared to stretch himself to enclose the thoughts of that particular patient, pain and all. That was why his H & P's were so life-giving. He absorbed his patients into his deepest thoughts. They never forgot him. This is what we must do with James, only we will seek to take his thoughts, without his body."

The sun was setting into a dim dusky rose twilight. I started to get up and then noticed the light seemed to be flickering. I plopped down in the chair.

"Bill, it seems to be flickering."

"What's flickering?"

"The air, over the bed. The light is coming together there and flickering. It seems golden with other colors, brown and blue, laced across it – like vibrations."

"What shape?"

"I'm imagining it kind of round, about a foot across. It's changing all the time but squishy. It's edges are shooting out here and there like little flames, but they're in rhythm with each other. My God, let me count. They're alpha brain wave rhythms. I'm seeing him think."

Bill moved to James' bed. "Okay, I'm going to try something with James, and you tell me if anything changes. Are you really in there, James? See if the rhythm changes."

"I'm just imagining James' brain waves in the light. All we have been doing has been sitting around talking about how James is really here, but we haven't believed it. That is intensely irritating."

Bill said soothingly, "Your imagining is important. It's an inspiration to go ahead and prove somehow that James' mind is alive. We knew what James was thinking much of the time. We've worked with him for a very long time. It's similar to knowing his mind. I care about him as you do and his mind also lives in me."

Bill added, "Over the years the three of us have made a systematic practice of creating a virtual interior reality of each other's minds. The same thing happens when you become 'lost' in a novel. You are 'there' amidst an inner reality of people, places and times. It requires a bit of artistry to achieve this subjective quality. It is different from just imagining. It is like stretching oneself over another person's thinking."

"That's good. So when I say that I'm imagining James' mind, I mean that I'm in that mind of his that lives within myself. When we come here to the hospital we never think we're going to visit a mentally damaged person. We're looking forward with enthusiasm to continuing the virtual reality we started so many years ago."

Breakthrough

Bill and I were doing something about James. We puttered about setting up three stands, one on each side of James' bed and one directly in front of him.

I taped flash-card letters to the left frame, "James, your horizontal eye movements are smoother today. In Locked-in Syndrome prognosis that's a good sign. If you look left, it will mean that you want one of the letters on this frame. Then we will point to each letter, and you will signal the right one by fixing your eyes on it when we point to it. If you want a letter in the center group or right group just look that way."

A managerial looking young man with dark, shining hair came in. He looked as if he had just graduated from high school, but his white coat indicated that he was on the hospital staff.

He strode up to look at our work and tried to stifle a laugh, "How interesting. Good morning, Dr. Howell. Oh, Dr. Moore, I was in a number of your master classes two years ago. I'm Joseph Brown, if you remember. I'm a speech therapist assigned to Dr. Herrer. The regular therapist will be by later. I see what you're trying to do. Actually, I have this small transparent plastic panel, you see, with six groups of letters set into it, which I can see through as I point to the letters. Much more efficient don't your think?"

He took one elegant finger and pushed aside the frames I had set by James' bed to hold the letters. "If I can just get in here, I'll show you how we do it."

One hour later he rose to leave. "As I expected there is no apparent cognitive functioning – certainly no linguistic capacity. Nice to see you again, Doctor."

Bill said, "Leave the plastic panel."

"I've just demonstrated, there's no need for it."

"I suggest you leave it."

"Very well, Dr. Moore. I'll just report to the department head that it's in your care."

After he left I began slinking around putting our equipment back up, "I guess these young therapists don't think old fogies are able to operate their hi-tech plastic."

Bill picked up the plastic panel, "It is a little neater than our system. Why don't we try this ourselves, and use the big frame for James. I think there are more opportunities for confusion about whether James' mind is working or not than he was aware of."

Bill continued, "Look here, there are six groups of letters. At the top of the board there is one group on the left, one in the middle and one on the right. Sit in the chair here by James' head so he can participate too. Now here I am holding it in front of you, Pat. I will send you a message. Remember you can't move your head or anything but your eyes. Your face is expressionless like a corpse. Are you looking at this group of letters?"

"I'm looking at you, Bill."

"Well, look at the letters. Anyway, since you're being James, you can't talk. You can't look disgusted either. OK. Are you looking here where I'm pointing? If that's correct, blink your eyes. . . you blinked, so this is the correct group."

I am getting frustrated. "Sometimes a blink is just a blink, Bill. I can't keep from blinking. Neither can James. Also with no facial muscle connections, he can't make an exaggerated blink. It's just his eyelid muscles that he has some control of. But no one has much control of blinks; they're mostly involuntary. Controlled blinks, like winks, require other facial muscles. Try it."

I added, "Rather than blinking, let's stick with James looking without moving his eyes. That's what we started out to do. I hadn't realized how hard it would be to set up a communication system with James if he couldn't tell us when we were doing something stupid."

Bill pulled up a chair and faces me, "Well, how about looking here at a group of letters? All right, now you're looking at this group I'm pointing to, right? No, you're looking at another group.

Well which is it?"

"I know I'm not supposed to be speaking, Bill, but sometimes an eye movement is also just an eye movement. They are mostly involuntary like blinks. You will have to wait for a very deliberate, long stare, and I'll have to concentrate very hard to keep my eyes from being distracted. Also you're not centering the board exactly on my face. I don't think you can tell where I am looking very well otherwise. I can't imagine that James' mind, if he has one, can control his eyes as he did in the past. His eyes will probably have more involuntary movements than mine. I like our own system better than this plastic sheet. The distance between groups is larger. The truth is that I'm frustrated already. It must have been much worse for James when that speech therapist was zipping through this procedure. Let's just use our own stands."

Thirty minutes later Bill, and I (pretending to be James), had managed to decipher three letters: Y O U....with misunderstandings of letters that hadn't been meant in between. We were both hot, sweaty and irritated.

I stood up over James and took my coat off. "James, let's do it. Bill, you handle the board and I'll write down the letters."

James' eyes seemed to be focused on me, then they shifted way over to the left away from the stands.

"Come on James, look at the board. We can do it – do something anyway even if the message is fragmentary."

After a struggle we did get a word, T H E. We celebrated with a couple of Cokes. James, of course, can't swallow. His body is getting its food through a tube.

For a moment I was overwhelmed with the reality of James' condition. Then trying to clear my throat, I said, "Well, let's continue. I am expecting something breathtaking from your mind."

The next letter is R (road? race?)

The next is M. I thought, "Ah, the mind of James, the Jungian world authority on dreams, has some fabulous insight on rapid eye movements in sleep but has left out the E. He means REM."

The next letter is O. The next is S; the next T.

"Bill, if you leave out the R as being a mistake, you have T H E (R) M O S T. Let's go for it."

The next letter is A; the next T.

"All right! T H E   M O S T   A T. The most at....where are the most at, James? Tell us."

James' eyes rest on me for a moment, then slide off to the left.

"He couldn't finish the sentence, Bill. Maybe it never was a sentence – just nonsense. He was probably tired out. I certainly am. I have to go and I know you do too."

Bill says, "James, we'll hit it again tomorrow," and leaves.

I noticed the sun would soon be down and stayed by the bed with my hand on James' forehead, thinking he might have some feeling there. I felt depressed and disheartened. All three of us had a lot riding on this. We were running out of time before James was condemned to death.

I sat down in the chair and watched the light turn to a dusky rose. Everything went out. There was only darkness.

Sometime later the door opened. The lights clicked on.

Susy came in, "What? Why Pat, what are you doing sitting over there in the corner? Have you been crying?"

"Just leaking a little, Susy. I'll see you tomorrow."

Stopping by the bed I said, "James, I'm sorry."

At home, tired and discouraged, I got into bed and fell into a hole of depression laced sleep.

Salvation

In the early morning hours the sound of a telephone ringing woke me. I groped for it.

Bill's voice was on the other end. "Not 'THE MOST AT!' Remember the R we dropped? Thermostat."

"THERMOSTAT! Of course, how obvious. How could I have been so stupid?"

Bill says, "We were tired and trying too hard."

"Do you remember, Bill? There was a thermostat on the wall to James' left. Even though his head couldn't move, he could just have seen it if his eyes were rolling."

I continued, "When I stood up to take my coat off I was right in front of his face. He would have seen how hot and sweaty I was. He sent 'thermostat,' then he looked at me and then at the thermostat – a clear, logical impeccable message. He was concerned, first, about my comfort. How like him. I'm the one with the cognitive deficits, not James."

Bill answers, "I expect James was angry with us. We failed him. He is probably very depressed."

I dialed Susy at the hospital, "Susy, hallelujah! I have a message for James."

"Pat, it's five o'clock in the morning. Are you all right?"

"I'm fine – sorry to wake you, but please go over to James' bed, be sure he's looking at you and say one word to him, 'thermostat.' Maybe he'll understand. I'll see you tomorrow and explain. Goodnight."

In the hospital later in the morning I spill some champagne on James' forehead, "I'm drinking this toast for you."

Bill, Susy and I clinked glasses and drink the champagne to celebrate James' message.

I poured some champagne down the thermostat. "We want you to join the party too."

Bill takes the bottle and says, "Let's remember that we have received only one word from James so far, and we didn't handle that one very well. If James doesn't send a strong clear message that he wants to live, they will find an opportunity to let him die. James can't swallow. You know he will have to have a tracheotomy almost immediately to seal off his mouth and throat from his lungs. He has to swallow in order to get the secretions in his mouth to drain into his stomach instead of his lungs. They will bypass the opening into his lungs and send secretions to the stomach. His body will certainly die without the tracheotomy, and the operation would be a perfect opportunity to let him die painlessly."

Bill bends over to look into James' eyes, "We have to get the transmission of a complete sentence down letter perfect. I suggest the sentence, 'I want to live.' That would be definite and something we could handle without a fatal mistake. Also if your eye movements don't work out perfectly, I can fudge a little since I know what you're going to say."

I set up the panels. "Let's do it. First, though l am going to tape on these two additions I made this morning, SPACE, to make the end of the word clear and PERIOD, to make the end of the message clear. Given a few days to practice, we will do it."

The door banged open and another speech therapist entered, two interns brought up the rear.

Bill was standing in the middle of the room holding the bottle of champagne in one hand with his mouth open.

Bill put the champagne bottle down, "This is not a good day to question Dr. Hall."

The speech therapist said in disgust, "No alcohol in the hospital, as you know." Then he hunched forward to peer at James' dead expressionless face. The two interns were huddled near the door looking apprehensive. This had the macabre atmosphere of putting a dead man on trial.

Bill cut in smoothly, "I suggest that we allow Dr. Hall to transmit a message on these panels we have here."

The therapist said, "I have been authorized to make a final determination here. Why don't we use the plastic spell board approved by my department. The question is 'Do you want to live?'" He thrust it in front of James' face.

I protested, "Those groups of letters are too close together for the control Dr. Hall has of his eye movements."

Bill moved to the therapist's side with the pointer, "Good. You hold the board, and I will use the pointer. Is this the group of letters you are looking at James? Good, now is this letter to which I am pointing the one you want?" James' eyes were floating around as he blinked. "No. This one? No. How about this one?" For a second James' eyes seemed to focus. "Yes, it is the letter I."

I picked up the pad and wrote down *I* then a space – James was getting it even with the little plastic spell board.

The next letter was *D*. The message was supposed to be *I want to live*.

I was thinking, "Why doesn't Bill fake it, help James to stay with the message? Yes, Bill is trying to suggest *W* but James keeps bringing him back to *D*. This is not the time to get confused, James."

The next letter was *E*.

The next letter was *M*, then *A. I DEMA* thirty minutes on five letters already. Time is running out.

Then *N*, then *D. I D E M A N D*. Come on James, don't try to be smart about this.

Then *T* and *O*. Then *L* and *I* and *V* and *E. I D E M A N D T O L I V E*

But more letters were coming, an *A*, an *S*, an *S*.

The next letter was an *H*, then and *O* and an *L . . .*

The therapist dropped the board.

Bill picked it up, "Let's see what the next letter is." *E. I D E M A N D T O L I V E A S S H O L E*

I shouted, "He has risen. Hallelujah!"

The two interns in the corner were breaking up. They left the room, talking as they went down the hall. This story will be told many times around the hospital before the day is over. The speech therapist sidled out the door.

Bill, Susy and I finished the champagne, and laughing and crying, talked to our beloved James.

IV

Patton Measures James

Locked In To Life

The Ouija/spellboard

Now James could finally communicate with us directly and tell us what had been happening in his mind. James had his plastic spellboard going twenty-four hours a day and was driving everyone crazy.

Susy, Bill, and I could all talk to James now, no matter how slowly or laboriously or how incomplete the conversations might be.

James wanted to do nothing but communicate constantly. I dropped the transparent plastic spelling board on James' bed and rubbed my sore hands. I hadn't yet made the transition from believing James' mind was functioning to being hit in the face with the reality of it.

"I'm exhausted, Susy. How about you?"

"I'm fine. Shall I read it now?"

But there was a quaver in her voice and a droop to her soft shoulders. She had been writing down the letters as I called them out. James had been driving everyone hard since we had discovered the plastic spelling board worked as well as our large frames. It had become a ouija/spellboard that communicated with a non-locatable ghost. It was easy to make mistakes. Spelling out the words letter by slow letter was laborious. Poor Susy — we had released a monstrous insatiable spirit which preyed upon her and gave her no rest.

Everything was the same, the morgue-like room, the cold, unmoving "corpse" on the bed; yet everything was amazingly different. An electric current of knowledge that James' mind was alive crackled through the air. Only now could we truly feel the burden we have all been under, trying to believe that he was still here without any real evidence.

I sighed. "Don't read it aloud, Susy. It will be more demands on us, no doubt. Let me read it to myself."

Susy reluctantly handed over her husband's message looking as though she wasn't sure she could trust me with it.

I've been thinking twenty-four hours a day since stroke. afraid not to. mind unraveled when didn't.

didn't see much at first but could soon hear everything. when U said something I would reply, no one heard.

repeating conversations to myself kept mind together.

must get this down. important. U three must get together and remember what U've said. I will tell U what U said, before U tell me. Then will tell what I was thinking at that time. I remember all. whole thing validated.

This was like getting messages from someone who had "passed over." Who is it? Who is communicating?

Bill came in. His solid presence seemed to cast stability and reassurance over the hospital room and the still body on the bed. I handed him the message from James.

Then Ouija/spellboard spelled out another message to Susy.

here is what I was thinking from the time of the stroke. silence. blackness. not breathing. touch. nothing to touch. up or down. nothing to feel. where are legs, hands. nothing to feel. no pain nothing to feel with. senses gone. dead. hear sounds with no source can see. not clearly. ceiling. slides past. fuzzy. can't focus. whiteness. white fuzziness is this death?

exactly what I thought. kept repeating it.

I was thinking, beneath a surface, and higher self is above.

no! don't want to die. want Susy.

I may be dead yet I exist.

know I am. unraveling mind spinning about a calm, certain center of myself. can't believe this. spent my life as a Jungian analyst seeking knowledge of life and death, and now I'm somewhere between life and death.

I am. how exciting. wait until I tell....but how can I tell?

We know.

no body-feelings to get confused with mental thoughts. my consciousness pure. no body.

U two thought U were so smart. from beginning U were trying to think like me so my own damaged thinking might be stimulated. well weren't U making fools of urselves?

let me tell U my thinking was just fine.

Bill and I had to agree that was essentially what we remembered.

also I'll have to admit that U did affect my thinking. my thinking could resonate with Urs. Our vibrations matched colors — blue to perfect blue, with purples matching and soft colors of red. thank U. it was big help.

wait, I know that I exist. perhaps I am already in the world of subjective reality. white walls, hospital waiting room. I remember. I was having a stroke. I knew I was dying.

how little I count, death could merely be a transition to life. without input from my body I am already in eternity.

am I linked to some other plane? am I part of a particular 'higher' self? is there a God?

is it possible that some part of me has survived death. but what part? my ego? no, not ego. know I exist. know thinking!

how does this death experience fit in? is this really happening or is it the product of a brain under severe stress?

how beautiful! I am hovering over my brain reading out those modules of brain cells that are open. what if this is another dimension?

to prove it will now tell U what U were saying.

his exact words. Pat said I'm like a drowning man holding on to life preserver. right?

I plopped down in the easy chair and closed my eyes. What had I said? Yet the phrase about the life preserver rang in my memory. Yes. I had said James was like a drowning man holding on to a life preserver.

I couldn't associate the mental power with this apparently dead body. So I said to the air around James' bed "How is it possible for you to remember every chance remark?"

Then the Ouija/spellboard replied,

what see is white haze. but mind works. all I had to do was remember and repeat what heard.

while Pat was visiting me, had difficulty understanding. trouble is don't hear sounds the way I remember hearing them. wait. don't have body reality. hadn't realized before that sounds heard in my mind were also vibrating in body. without body they're ghost-sounds. pure concentration to keep them from fading out.

getting what little meaning I do because know both Pat and Bill so well.
have had years to build up representations of both Pat and Bill. could prob-
ably have conversations with both of them in imagination.

OK Pat, try this one. bet U can remember. were talking about me being
a round-bottomed set of russian dolls. poor taste. then tried to tell joke about
blonde. said U didn't remember hearing it.

I remembered talking about the set of Russian dolls, and the
joke. You could make a blonde's eyes sparkle by shining a flashlight in her ear. I said, "They're both very clear."

U had heard it before. remember told U about eight months ago. was not
communicating verbally with U, but I was apparently influencing Ur mind.

my thinking that joke did not 'cause' U to imagine it.

OK, I get it! this is what happened. when U tried to think in my mind
U subjectively created a mind so close to mine I was interacting with U.
matching the color vibrations of my thoughts with yours.

how possible? it isn't ESP; I'm one of the world's experts on that.
Extra Sensory Perception means an effect caused by an unknown kind of
perception. however, I was in tune with my mind in your mind.

I could remember "imagining" that James and I were communicating and James affirms that we were actually interacting
through knowing each other so well. It was not a mysterious
objective ray of perception as ESP speculates. "Good point
James."

The spellboard urged us on.

go back to when my colleagues met in my hospital room to plan how to
murder me. what I heard in different pontifications was: Kill! Kill!

now, going to tell you exactly what I was thinking then — word for word.
have to keep repeating or mind disintegrates.

tell them they're wrong Pat, before its too late. don't let them kill me!
God! don't let them kill me!

keep in mind I was thinking back then — not now.

that's it! care rather than kill! physicians must care for life rather than
kill life — especially for the mental life of the self. I thought had learned so
much about mind and self that I could tell U about it if I could just make
U hear. if I ever get stable control of my eyes, maybe.

I *may* have said and written things about being killed if I couldn't function. I didn't realize that I could be effectively non-functional — dead — and
still have all of my mind and my self. having my mental self is what being

truly functional means!

Pat, find that stupid paper I wrote and destroy it.

no I didn't mean to kill me. I didn't know how it would be. I take it back. listen, I take it back!

don't let these jerks pull the plug on my soul. I've got to get through to U. help! I'm about to be murdered. help! save me. help!

talk about interacting! I was fully interacting then.

Bill and I didn't have to confer, "All three of us were speaking off the same page on that one. It's good to feel that we were together even though we couldn't communicate."

I exclaim. "Then what we've really been discovering all this time is that the mind can do without a body."

Me. I'm the proof. Says Ouija\spellboard.

Bill said to the air, "Who are you besides a haunt, or a ghost, or a Ouija/spellboard that tires us all out?"

The spellboard answered.

why should I be tired? mind doesn't have to run body. mind has own energy.

I'm free. don't have physical resources I used to need in order to speak — lungs, voice box, tongue, lips, etc. — thousands of discrete physical operations just to say a word.

now all I have to do is focus my eyes. don't have a body input. have no body. none of the background noise of body. exist in an absolute body silence.

nothing but pure consciousness. have all the time there is. have absolutely nothing else to do.

A Message for Susy

James has been moved to a rehabilitation hospital. He had become an embarrassment where he was. Bill and I were together in his new hospital room. I was draped over a chair. Bill was standing beside James' bed with the Ouija/spellboard in hand. "James, I have noticed that you don't use your eyes to see, only to communicate with the spellboard."

right. very important. eyes not used to see. only to concentrate. all my mental ability into communicating. matter of life or death.

at first no sight or sound. not blackness. nothing. a void with nothing but my mind. then changed to white haze. a succession of white hospital ceilings. parts of walls. then could see ceilings as ceilings — grasp the 'ceiling.' parts of walls as walls when my eyes rolled, only sometimes upside down and sometimes right side up. not consistent patterns.

had to concentrate solely on thinking patterns or lose my mind. everything perceptual became a shimmery white haze again. hospital rooms have few perceptual features. the voices I heard were more understandable a more primitive orientation.

real question is would U recognize me as ghost if my voice were scrambled to prevent my using normal voice clues, what could I tell U on the phone to convince you that it was really me.

"What could convince me it was really you?" I answered, "Your language, of course, the way you use words. I can identify the way your mind works. Your thoughts are unique. They are the most characteristic thing about you That's how I would know it was you."

James continued.

telephones, TV, computers, books are all disembodied communication and interaction.

one day bed put in hall in awkward position. people ignored me. including nurse. having no people better than ones who ignore me. felt invisible. mind is the ability to elicit interaction from others.

after about five hours moved back into my room. realized how much the sense of physical existence depends upon people interaction. I find myself adjusting to my limitations.

I felt filled with foreboding, "Do you realize you were talking about your limitations, James? You are free of the limitations of your body now. You never used or needed your body anyway except for gourmet food and sex. This materialist hospital is getting to you."

Bill broke in, "I think Pat is right. You are approaching the awareness of a conflict of the mental and physical dimensions of experience."

Two nurses came in to pour a flask of liquid food into the tube that goes to James' intestines, change his smelly diapers, make his bed, and change his clothes.

When they left, I commented, "I notice that the only body maintenance activities I resent are the ones where the physical therapists pretend they are giving James back a body. Since they have to accept his mind. They can't stand it if he doesn't have a body."

Bill gave me a look.

James' ouija/spellboard explained his mind was changing.

mental existence nor pure when relating to people living in physical world. that pulls me towards my lost body. maybe the physical therapy I'm getting now will help. maybe I don't have to live as a ghost. don't you understand what it would mean to me to experience the life of the senses again? I have been accepting myself as a ghost for so long.

Bill left, and I began to stretch my legs, holding the spellboard for a last message.

wait! I want to tell you a little more. it's very important.

With a sigh I began to record James' eye movements again. The following is the result:

met Susy when I was thirteen. the prettiest girl I had ever seen. married when I was twenty-one. can't say that life was peaceful. was very immature. U know there have been other women, and I haven't supported Susy enough.

never wished to be married to anyone else. have something right. seems I am different from my history of myself, from person thought I was. betrayed her, while in my self always loving her.

wonder if my trouble with Susy has been immaturity on my part. fear of closeness. fear of being smothered. also feared with my mother. hard on Susy. don't want to live unless I can live with Susy. in first vision after stroke I asked to return to life in order to be with her. dying thoughts were literally of her.

My eyes watering, "That's beautiful, James. Have you told Susy this?"

no.

"Well, in God's name, why haven't you?"

when she's here with the board, it's too hard. I need a more intimate way.

"Well, look. I'll write it down here as part of today's report, and give it to her. Then she can read it by herself – like reading a book."

James writes.

that's good, Pat, like a book. we've been working on reconstructing the time I couldn't get through to U or her. she can sit down and relax with this. that's nice.

That night I went by Susy's house. She had begun staying home a little recently. As I walked down her entrance hall I remembered her as a young woman. She was slender with an ethereal beauty and large luminous eyes which dominated her face. Her eyes were truly windows to a sensitive and vulnerable soul. She was expecting a wonderful life married to this brilliant young man with whom she was so much in love.

I sighed for her as I walked into a living room piled high with recently arrived professional journals and reports.

Susy gestured helplessly, "Look, James would go through all this before you knew it. He could read a page at a glance, as you know. All I can do is just stack it up here. At least he's not here demanding that I do this and then do that. His friends would come over and I would be expected to wait on them and even run errands for them and some of them women, with that look in their eyes. Would you like a drink?"

I hastily declined.

Susy touches me tenderly, "Oh, I wasn't talking about you."

I handed her the note from James, "I just brought this by for you, Susy. I thought you might want to read it here by yourself."

I left feeling good.

We never spoke another word about the letter.

Imagined Mind

The reconstruction of the first weeks of James' uncommunicated thoughts in the hospital took seven weeks to express itself.

The burden of recording James' communications on the spellboard fell mostly on Susy. Bill and I had our practices to run, but we visited the hospital room as often as possible.

At any rate it was done. James had been pushing everyone. He had been obsessed with saving and recording his thoughts during the time he could not communicate. Everyone else had become obsessed too.

James' communications were now representing his current thoughts, rather than proving he had been thinking all along. Also he was now beginning to take time to produce more grammatical messages.

Barbara Hannah had an interesting theory. She believed that humankind did not intrinsically have a soul, but that it had the opportunity to construct a soul. It is important to be clear that she meant soul in the traditional sense, as that which is most vital in mankind. Barbara seemed to mean that one used imagination so forcefully that it acquired a reality of its own. Rather like imagining a brick with such forcefulness that one could stumble over it. She definitely seemed to assign some reality to imaginal constructions.

Her notion seemed to be that one enters active imagination and from that position constructs another mind that has a life of its own in a unique space, again of its own. Death of the physical body might leave the imaginal body untouched. One could then inhabit it.

All of this sounds preposterous from our usual way of thinking – everything that happens to us is caused. But if I believe we are all creators and that imagination, especially active imagination, is the way we create.

James had been on a mental high during this almost two-month period of reconstruction, his mind fizzing like champagne.

He was insatiable for contact with others. He claimed that they were his mental nourishment. It was only as he ate them that he became more real, mentally. People were either still unable to believe what had happened or were uncertain about the situation – so few people came by to see James. Those few were saints; they lighted up his life.

Telling the story of that time, I acquired an enriched dimension of its reality that was more true (as a musical note is true) than the original experience. The mental dimension seemed more real than the physical one. I had become disembodied myself to that extent.

An Inner World

I had a problem at the hospital that lasted late and afterwards, I thought I would go by James' room. He was able to communicate using all the letters grammatically now.

Susy, looking harassed says, "He spent all day getting me to write this for you," and handed me several sheets of paper. Here they are.

Let me give you an example of how I spend my nights. I was thinking what virtual world will I create tonight? Bill and Pat, I command you to enter my mind and for tonight become my virtual reality. Let's have one of our old meetings on the study of self.

I'll do it pretending it's at your house, Pat. I remember that we once discussed your work on rapid eye movements at your house. People's eyes move behind their closed eyelids when they're seeing things in their dreams. It's as though they were seeing material things when in fact the reality is not material at all but completely subjective – mental.

Now, I'm going to recreate everything at your material house that night in my mind. This will be my mental exercise to awaken my recalcitrant, moronic, neuronic cells. If the old cells are dead, other cells will just have to learn my mental commands. Get with it cells, I command you. For all of our sakes, I have to get control of my eyes.

OK, here we go. I am creating the reality of Pat and Bill in my thoughts regardless of their material existence elsewhere. I am composing the place, starting with the table. Pat's wife, Joan, always set a magnificent table for us. That will be my inspiration. Here now is my reality of a plate with three kinds of olives: green, ripe, and wrinkled oil-cured ones. There is also a plate with three kinds of sliced meats: roast beef, thickly sliced salmon, and smoked turkey that tastes like ham. Some kind of pickled herring is in a bowl, as is mayonnaise and coarsely ground mustard and bread! There are three kinds of bread, all chewy and home baked. The brown was my favorite. There was onion salad, which Bill especially likes. I am pleased to see cheeses and a plate of rumaki, a strong candidate for the world's best food. There are also chicken livers skewered by a toothpick with water chestnuts. They are each wrapped in bacon and lightly broiled.

I fill a plate in my imagination and settle into one of the wing-backed chairs for some good conversation. Soon we are hard at it, punctuated by bites of good food. I know that I am relying on images of Pat and Bill built up in my mind over many years of conversations with them. But the images have a life of their own. In this case they have a life of their own even down to the color of Bill's socks.

Suddenly the image of Pat says something about books that startles me. I am now possessed by a subjectively real Pat living within me and not mere fantasy as the food seems to have been.

This Pat and Bill are different than the real Pat and Bill. But are they real? The possible reality of sympathetic magic (what you think becomes real) goes very far back in mankind's belief, at least as far back as the old kingdom of ancient Egypt, and that's pretty far back. These images of Pat and Bill are virtually alive. They can surprise me like the real Pat and Bill. Moreover, they seem to grow over time just like the real Pat and Bill. Was this what Pat meant in his book about characters in novels having a mental reality more real than our material casual acquaintances? In the mind we approach each other, mutually dedicated to an interior creation bigger than either of them alone. We are in sacred precincts when we approach the other.

I'm wandering and am about to lose touch with this dinner with Pat and Bill. Too bad, my friends, that your so-called real selves can't participate.

Bill sits in one of the wing-backed chairs; Pat, stretches himself out like a cat along the couch.

"Well," begins Pat, "I am participating. It seems to me that there is a core of being before there is a self. Babies have it. Self is a story we tell ourselves about ourselves."

"Oh, Pat," says Bill, attacking a slice of corned beef with his fork. "I think it's power again. The ego is just another way of talking about the ego's power drive. It cannot control everything, you see, but it tries!"

The image of me breaks in: "I think there are two things — the ego and where it identifies itself. It may identify with power or it may not. But the bare bones of the ego is just awareness."

It's interesting that this Pat and this Bill are able to surprise me even more than active imagination or a dream. It's the personality, that surprises me. Maybe I am a guinea pig in an experiment of the nature of self.

I've just seen that the disembodied selves of Bill and Pat can be alive and real. There was one me at this dinner both creating it and living it – and living also with my creations of Bill and Pat.

I'm using interactions with you two to focus my mind – Will I ever get home again? I want to see my dog. I don't sleep anymore. If I ever let my mental focus waver, my mind seems to begin to unravel. I'm afraid my very self might dissolve into the universal mind. I'm going to keep telling myself my stories like this over and over again.

I had sat down to read this in the easy chair by his bed with my feet propped up on his bed covers. "I gather you must have been living a virtual life like this all the time we couldn't communicate with you."

Ouija/spellboard, *Yes, you understood. This is a new way of living.*

I put the board down before he could say anything more and left for the day.

Do Ghosts Have IQ's?

Two days later I was on my way up to James' room when my old friend Rachael Skouras from the hospital's mental health department caught me in the hall. Rachael was slim and had a Mediterranean-complexion. She invited me into her office.

She also had chutzpah. As she sat down behind her desk, she said, "The last few weeks, I've been hearing stories around the hospital about Dr. Hall. Is there any validity to them?"

"There sure as hell is."

I told her how James saved his own life by summoning up the primitive eye control necessary to communicate. They hadn't been able to stop him since.

Rachael's eyes brighten with interest, "Are you saying that a fragment of a brain is actually producing some activity one could call mentation? I could imagine short incoherent statements. But you certainly can't expect me to believe that the self survived."

"I'm not sure who or where self is. But the messages we are getting are as coherent and closely reasoned as any you are ever likely to see. His existence is recognizably James' self. He's even quoting references with name, volume, and date, for the points he is making."

Leaning back in her chair Dr. Skouras asks, "Could you test him for the extent of his cognitive deficits?"

"There are no cognitive deficits. Let me put it into perspective this way: A person whose mind is totally integrated with his body can be a glorious human being of great value. But if that person's body were removed, that integrated person would have no mind. That is your medical experience, right? It is Dr. Herrer's experi-

79

ence. I don't blame him for being unable to believe that James' mind exists."

I added, "But think of someone like James who has spent his life as a mental being, along with his physical lusts. He had a Buddha body. You could sit his body in a chair and it would stay there regardless of where his mind was. Believe me, I know. I've worked with him and Bill Moore for years on a study of just this kind of situation – mind beyond body. James has been able to hold his mind together and preserve it. I expect you at least to be open to the possibility, Rachael."

She leans forward, a little tense. "If I accept that possibility, I accept the further possibility that some of those silent bodies hooked up to tubes here in the hospital are prisons for functioning minds. When I pause near those beds to check vital signs, do you want me to accept that those minds are crying out to me, pleading to be heard? Do you want me to live with the guilt of having abandoned even one or two people in their useless bodies because I didn't have time to try to establish communication with their existing minds somehow?"

"Yes."

"You can go to hell. Can't you understand how frightening it is for a doctor to face a mind without a body? I was starting to ask if you could adapt some cognitive testing protocols to his condition, but now I'm afraid to ask."

But she smiled with affection. She was afraid, but she wanted to know the truth, "Can you do it?"

"Yes."

"Can you say anything other than yes?'

"Yes. I will give him the Wechsler Adult Intelligence Scale. How do you like that."

"You're crazy. First it's a timed test. Second, it requires physical movement, like putting a physical puzzle together. He can't do it."

I slapped a bill on her desk, "If you feel that way, you just cover that ten spot."

She rummaged around in her purse for a bill and pounds it down on top of mine, saying "I'll keep the money."

"However, I will agree that timing only be applied to a 'Yes' or

'No.' then he can spell out the answer untimed. If he's wrong he fails the question."

I couldn't time the test, but I thought I could handle the physical requirements. This was the only way to do it – with only minor deviations from standard testing procedures. Rachael would make a formidable ally if I could pull it off.

As I entered James' room, the low sun has cast an amber light across the floor. Where was the aura that once hovered over James' bed? It seemed as though that happened in another time and place – a place of other dimensions, of possibilities beyond this world.

"James, I've got a great idea. I know you must have had a Wechsler Adult Intelligence Scale done in medical school, right?"

Ouija/spellboard, *Yes. 135.*

"Okay, I will administer the Wechsler IQ using the old WAIS form you would have been given. That way, using the same instrument, we can demonstrate how well you are thinking. Also, I've got a kind of bet about your mental condition with Rachael Skouras. Even she can't really grasp that you have a fully functioning mind. I'm going to run by the office. I'm sure I put the old WAIS kit in the closet there instead of throwing it away when the new version came out. Be back soon."

The truth was that everyone had cognitive deficits. Just getting up in the morning leaves most of us with cognitive deficits until we've had our coffee and breakfast. I could be getting myself into big trouble trying to compare James' WAIS scores when he was a feisty young medical student immersed in an environment of highly competitive tests with this entity communicating slowly and painfully through barely controlled eye movements. Not only were his face and body immobile, even those muscles that give expression around his eyes are frozen – the only control he has is the slow uncertain movements of the eyeballs themselves.

Because the WAIS, was a timed test, James' mental self would be at a terrible disadvantage. There were ways to level the playing field somewhat. To comply with the timing requirement, James could signal when he knew the answer. That would be timed. And then he could spell out the answer untimed. That answer must be correct.

Any adjustments made must be demonstrably and exhaustively justified with the testing protocol or no one would believe the results. On the other hand James might do so poorly that the results couldn't even be scored. It couldn't be hidden if it was bad; I was committed to the truth. If I hadn't thought that James' mind was confident, I would have talked her into a less dramatic cognitive test.

We would find out.

The Wechsler Adult Intelligence Scale

I returned to James with my testing kit in hand. Susy posted a "No Admittance Testing in Progress" sign on the door.

With some trepidation, I began. My hopes were immediately dashed during the first subtest. This subtest was about information. Halfway through it was a question asking for a date. James' eyes didn't give the up and down movement which signifies that he knew the answer.

"Don't you know it, for Christ's sake?"

No.

His answer is in the time limit. If it had been "yes," then he could have spelled it out untimed.

Then I realized that I didn't know it either. Fortunately, I had the answers in front of me.

I said, "So you made a mistake."

One plus to giving this IQ test to a disembodied spirit was that the disembodied spirit couldn't turn his head to see the diagnostician looking up the answers.

But that is the only one James missed, getting 28 correct answers out of 29 questions. In the comprehension of words subtest he got all the questions right. Arithmetic did not go as well. The similarities subtest was tricky. But he almost got a perfect score. He scored perfectly on vocabulary, which I expected.

The Performance part of the IQ was unfair to James. The object assembly subtest was a timed completion of a jigsaw puzzle. I held up the pieces one by one in front of his face. To do this he had to remember each piece in his mind while he moved them around mentally. He was timed on how long it took to tell the object the pieces would make. Then he had all the time it took to tell how to put the pieces together. This didn't follow the rules of the test, but it seemed an acceptable compromise.

James did poorly on the performance tests. Ghosts don't perform very well materially. As it turned out, an hour's test took two days to complete. I had tried to be exhaustive, and I was exhausted. James was fine; he wanted to keep communicating.

"I'm sorry, James. I must retire and score this test," I said, "It's very uneven. I can't guess now how it will turn out."

I dawdled getting to the hospital the next day. I had scored the test, rethought the method of administering it, checked it for internal consistencies, and was now thinking about how to put it to Rachael. I decided to let her score the raw results herself. I stopped by Rachael Skoura's office.

She looked up from some files, "Has it ever occurred to you to call before coming by?"

"Yes. No, not really. Rachael, I'm worried about how to break these IQ test results to James. Giving the Wechsler Adult Intelligence Quota to disembodied minds is not exactly standard procedure."

Rachael looked concerned, "Oh, so you've done it. I'll have to place it in the hospital files, you know. Let me see it."

I handed her the file of James' test results, but I held back the score calculation. She opened it, skimmed the results and frowned a terrible frown. I had known she would.

She pulled a chair up to her side of the desk, "Sit down. You say this is a test of a disembodied mind. We are going to go over this item by item."

We went over the verbal section. She questioned and fought me on everything. But the verbal is straightforward. I had taken his answers off the Ouija/spellboard and written them down exactly as they came off.

"Look," she said, "all these words. How do you prove they weren't some other word? How do you prove it's James in the first place?"

"Look, Rachael," I said, "I don't know where the entity is who is spelling, but it sure as hell sounds like James. Also getting letters correctly is very difficult with this spellboard, but I am being fanatically precise in putting it down just as it happens. The ambiguity is in the process, not in James. See, here where he gives an answer in the similarity subtest. The spellboard gives me the answer. I don't extrapolate and put down this letter exactly. That's all."

Rachael takes my hand, "Calm down, don't shout. Doubting is my job. But I'll O.K. this part as valid."

"Aargh!"

"Now let's go on to the physical part. Well, this is a complete mess. How can a paralyzed body....Oh, I see. He's telling you what to do."

"Well, what did you expect, Rachael?"

I unzipped the test kit and took out some cartoon pictures, "Look I had to hold each of these in front of his face. His mind would have to remember them all, create a synopsis in the time limit and then take an hour, still remembering them, to communicate the proper story to me."

I started holding the cartoon pictures up. "You try it."

Rachael starts laughing. "All right, put them away. I concede."

I hide a smile.

By the time we finished the whole thing, we were tired and snapping at each other.

Rachael slacked back in her chair. Then I suggest she score it herself. She did and added it all up. Then it hit her, "But he's made 135 even with those handicaps. That is impossible! He can't be operating at such a high mental level."

We looked at each other. I let my smile break through. Then she jumps up, "You rat! You tricked me. If you had showed me the score first I would never have believed you."

I laughed, "You'll have to certify it now, Rachael, for the hospital records."

Rachael was happy about this. I mean she really was. After rummaging in her purse she walked with me to the door. She pushed me into the hall, "You win. Here's your money. Go ahead and tell James now. I'll certify it – not standard but valid."

Trying to enter the hospital room unobtrusively, I listened to Bill saying he was leaving as soon as he could get rid of the Ouija/spellboard. We don't address ourselves directly to James' frozen body anymore, but rather to the air around it as though seeking the spirit that must be there.

"If you can stay just a moment Bill, I have the IQ score." Moving up to James' bed, "It doesn't seem possible, James, but you scored the same as you did when you were in medical school."

Bill dropped the Ouija/spellboard to the floor.

"The differences are well within the range of the built-in error of the test. But the point is that no one will be able to continue talking about cognitive deficits. This shows that even though a major portion of your brain cells are dysfunctional, your mind is just as good as it ever was. How you're holding your disembodied self together, how your immaterial mind can express itself so precisely through your eyes. I simply don't understand. I don't know what the medium is in which you exist or where it is, but our scientific colleagues are going to have to come to terms with this. We have established by objective testing the extent of your mental functioning."

Bill gets excited, "This is fabulous, unbelievable!" He lingers over "unbelievable" and looks at me suspiciously.

"Cut it out, Bill. I've been over the test results and my procedures with Rachael Skouras. She says that while some of my procedures would not have been acceptable in a normal test setting, she is convinced that the results reflect a valid IQ score."

With these IQ test results there was no doubt that we would be able to ask a local foundation to pay for a computer. There was a computer that could type with light focused from a person's eyes. It had a board with the alphabet on it like the spellboard, but one activated it by light reflecting from looking at the letter he wanted. It was expensive, but the Institute Board had already approved a study of James' case. James is the best research subject the project could possibly find.

Patton Howell   James Hall

V

Patton's Exit

Locked In To Life

Temptations

Since Rachel Skouras forced the hospital to accept James' unbelievable IQ score, he was being treated like a real person all day. Strapped up in his wheelchair he was just as corpse-like as ever, but people treated him as though he was alive much more than they did when he was in bed. His reaction mirrored this new acceptance. He now thought of himself as more embodied. He also felt more sharply the negative deficits of being disembodied rather than the positive mental differences of living completely in a subjective dimension.

A therapist bustled in. He was young, bursting with health and muscles. It seemed an intolerable intrusion of physicality into our spiritual haven. "I'll have to ask you all to leave during my physical therapy session. After a preliminary routine he will be down in the therapy room."

I said, "You must be the man from Porlock."

"No," he says, "I'm not from Porlock, wherever that is. What are you talking about?"

"There is a story about an English poet, Coleridge, who was writing a poem when a man from Porlock called on him. Coleridge could never get his poem going again after the interruption. We've been exercising James' mind, and you've come in to exercise his body. You might say that we're each from Porlock, in relation to the other."

The young man grins, "This is the place where we take care of bodies; so you must be the one from Porlock."

They leave. I found my treatment of the young man the object of Bill's censorious gaze.

The next day I asked James how the physical therapy went.

Therapist found me boring. Talked about exercises being monotonous but necessary. Complained room too cold. Complained about not having another place to see me. Next room too noisy. The therapy room had balloons painted on the walls. When I could see them I handled my boredom by counting them. Are there 42 or 44? I kept finding new ones that I had not counted. I am not as incompetent as that sounds – balloons indeed! – but I could seldom see all the three walls. I had to be on guard against subtle negative suggestions, though unconscious, from the therapist, 'This is hard' he would say, 'but we'll never know if you can do it unless we try.'

Lucky to be alive. But am off balance about the reality of mind vs body. Dissatisfied physically keeps me always trying to reach beyond my mind. Where and what am I?

Having finite physical limitations, yet trying to reach beyond them has always been a part of the human condition. No different than anybody else. I experienced my mental reality as having no limitations. I am still trying to find body. Terms are more stark for me. Will regain my lost body.

I felt impatient, things are changing. The hospital routine was changing. James was changing. I can feel him preparing to say good-bye to the boundless mental existence where he has been. Even though he is still disembodied, he is feeling more a part of the physical world. There's a conflict looming.

I knew that Susy agreed with James. She wanted to get the body she loved back and functioning. I couldn't disagree with her wish, but I was afraid the wish wouldn't come true. I kept my mouth shut about this topic when I was with Susy.

As is often the case with bureaucracies, the hospital had gone from one extreme to the other. Instead of ignoring James, someone now seemed to be coming in every few minutes to physically rehabilitate him in some way. But while he could carve new very limited neural channels for his mind, too much of his brain was gone for him to overcome his quadriplegia. The problem was how the hospital treated James' lost body. Since the IQ test, the attitude seemed to be, "If we can't avoid the existence of Dr. Hall's mind, then we must have a body to go with it." It was as though the existence of a mind without a body was an unthinkable, insupportable obscenity.

I realized that my own inner boiling of resentment at these

intrusions of the physical therapy program into James' mind revealed my own obsession.

I told Bill, "I'm trying to save his mind. Why are they fooling around with his unnecessary body? There is a mind, a new kind of disembodied self in the universe, that cannot be buried with the body. Like air it will rise up and cannot be stopped, but must rise up and up and go ....where? To the future perhaps – road signs to the human future. Can we call it a mind without a body? Like gravity, I know it does exist even if I cannot say how it exists, even if, like gravity, I cannot touch or feel or see it. The only way I know it is through the material signs of its immaterial existence. James is being seduced into believing that the only way his mind can exist is to find its lost body."

An Electronic Body

The local foundation finally approved the computer operated by looking at the alphabet. Everybody wanted to push for its early delivery. Then James' mind would be in control. He wouldn't have to depend on someone holding the spellboard in his face.

It was hard for the foundation to deliver the computer. It was the result of the highest level of research technology. They were only made one at a time. Even after the negotiations were completed, there was another wait while it was shipped from Pittsburgh. Now was the big day. I wheeled James into the Speech Department, checked with the secretary that he had an appointment there. The Ouija/spellboard, his lifeline of communication, was still in the pack on the back handles of his chair.

In a few minutes Nancy, the communications specialist, came out of her windowless office to get us. On her desk was what looked like a new briefcase. She opened it up to reveal a portable computer and a board with letters on it. The entire alphabet was arranged as on a typewriter keyboard. With this computer James could initiate interactions without waiting for someone to pick up the spellboard. He could write all day by himself without any help from anyone. He could carry on a conversation with it. The computer could even speak words, but what it said was often pronounced so badly that it was not understandable. However, people could read the message as it was typed out. That was the real communication.

The End of Patton's Story

I have been telling the story of James. Now I can hand it over to James himself. It had been the story of a man who lost his body and yet still lived. Now he demanded to tell his story himself. For the time being, at least, he fired me, who had been validating the happenings you have read.

In all of human tradition there is an implied trade-off: "I will give my soul's life to have more body-life" or "I will give my body's life to have more soul-life." Such choices are worth paying attention to because you are making them every day, whether you know it or not.

Living without a body brings into question our basic assumptions about life. "What is body?" "What is living?" "Do I value myself only as body or am I something more?"

What is a "self?" Self implies a unique, irreplaceable entity. What would be the point of existence if you had no self? It is true that your body, like your fingerprints, is unique. Mental self is also unique.

The deepest human fears are usually about such fundamental and unanswered questions as, "Who am I?" "What is the meaning of my mind, of my body?" "What is death?"

Imagine an empty wooden casket sitting beside a hole where two men are digging. "We're sending Joe here back to Missouri," they say. "Family wants him there." They are shoveling black dirt in the casket.

"But this is just...."

"That's Joe," says one of the diggers. "What did you think he would look like? Look there! See that finger bone? They're scattered all through this dirt."

"How long has he been....?"

"About 10 years."

Flesh into dirt by 10 years. What is the experience of death as a handful of dirt?

If we seek silence and listen, we will find the innate knowledge that our bodies must perish. We know instinctively that natural life can grow and change only through the death of our bodies. We know that there is a time for our bodies to die. We know our bodies are the material messengers of a non-physical message. That message is not the body's genes. Twins (or clones) have the same genes, but different selves. That message is a mental message of self. Surely there is a mental self which exists beyond bodily self?

Results of experiments in the psychophysiology of aging show that people at age 60 begin to think about what it means to be living after 85. They get uncomfortable imagining living past 95, and they get irritated with the suggestion they might be alive beyond 100. Life at 150 is felt to be out of time. Such a lifespan feels like immortality to most people. The most frequent comment has been, "Well, what would I do if I were really old? What kind of life would I have at that age?"

We tend to get nervous as we approach the possibility of the mind locked in a disintegrating body. We start thinking in terms of conditions. We don't say, "I'll do anything, put up with any hardship, to live a long time." Rather we say, "I might be willing to live to be 95, if I felt good." But such criteria are all physical ones.

The kind of immortality we are referring to is the immortality of mind. But how much loss of body function are you willing to put up with in order to live longer mentally? This implies that there is an insubstantial immaterial you, a personal mind that must exist if body is to have any meaning.

The origin of this concept in Western culture has been the myth of the soul, in particular the myth of Faustus who sold his soul to the devil. Thereafter he found that without his soul, his body's life was meaningless. We still have stories – mostly jokes – in which the devil appears and says, "Sell me your soul, I will give you...."

What if there could be a personal self beyond a body? Isn't

that what people have thought of as mind? It is ancient wisdom, but it has suffered from being associated with religion. Science and religion have always been at war. Science has sent spaceships to heaven and discovered no souls with halos and wings. Science has successfully debunked the special creation of man in the Garden of Eden. In the midst of its rightful victories in the war with religion, science has left unexamined the question of a self beyond the body – of James.

Locked In To Life

VI

James' Story

Locked In To Life

I'm in Charge

I hope the preceding helped prepare you for me. This is James Hall. It's been five years since my stroke. I am writing this time on my own computer. This must be clearly understood. I can now spell and punctuate properly. I'm in charge. This is my story to tell, and I am going to tell it without having to rely on someone interpreting for me on the spellboard. Words will not appear here unless I write them. My mind is using a beam of light reflected from my eyes to type these words. My mind has a new body, an electronic computer. I am embodied in a computer. I must make you understand. These typed words are me. They are all the face, voice, hands, and body that I have. These words are my material existence. How can I let you know how much it means to once again have a material existence? I gladly gave up the freedom of soul I found when I was unbound from time.

In any case I had been waiting to talk to Pat about our writing a book together about my experiences. I felt that since he had won that national literary award for his book *Beyond Literacy*, the year before that he would have an idea about how to approach it. He said there was no problem with writing our book.

I miss seeing Pat. We had an argument. I regret it and I find myself dwelling on it now that he's left on a lecture tour.

When he came in that day, he had said, "Well, hi ol' friend."

It's good to see you. I feel a little more embodied this week, I typed.

"Very nice," he said, but something in his face said otherwise. He paused a long while, seemingly in thought, then said, "You know, the more you are embodied, the more you are selfish."

To hell with you!

"You don't have to get upset about it! Think back to before your stroke. Your direct interactions with others were filled with deceit. None of us with body needs can afford to be absolutely truthful. It's a power game based on body not on mind. During your locked-in time you were just happy to be mentally alive, your interactions with others were free. No more need to play the power game for your body. You know, as your mind becomes more embodied – even being computerized is a kind of embodiment – it also becomes bitchier."

I'm not even sure 'bitchier' is a word.

"You know what I mean!" he shouted, very unlike his usual laid-back tone.

Goodbye!

"Goodbye!" said Pat, and he left.

I felt crappy. I hadn't really wanted him to leave when I printed Goodbye. I had never argued in anger with Pat before.

The next day when Pat came to visit, I told him that he was right – that I did seem to get more selfish the more embodied I was.

"Thank you," he said. "It fits right in!"

With what? I asked, genuinely bewildered.

"Why, with my view of the body-mind relationship, of course! You see, at its base self-centeredness rests upon the body, on its need to maintain itself. Without the body, the mind is free to be itself!"

Don't get carried away.

"Sorry. Look at it this way. The needs of the body – water, temperature, food – things like that would be meaningless to the mind unless it had always thought of itself as identified with the body; in that case the body's needs would seem to be its needs, too. Although they wouldn't really be. See?"

I didn't want to admit that Pat was right. But, my God, I had to. I seem to have these necessary confessions to make to Pat and Bill.

My mind survives as long as I can keep thinking. It is not threatened with the minute-by-minute needs of the body. In fact it's quite clear to me now that the more I have bought into the illusion of embodiment presented by my physical therapy, the more selfish I've become.

I wrote, *My physical therapy is now centered on the survival of a body that I can't feel physically. I know all this, yet I've been seduced by all of this physical therapy. I've created an imaginary body with selfish body needs. Let's talk more about this selfishness thing.*

Pat seemed pleased that I thought his observation was correct."Say, that's important. Maybe that's why meditation makes one more selfless – or non-attached as the Buddhists would say."

I wrote, *What would be complete disembodiment? Bodily death, I suppose. Maybe at our bodies' death we become completely unselfish, completely at one with everything.*

"There are a lot of people that I wouldn't care to be at one with," Pat said.

I could tell he was not in the mood for serious conversation.

Me too, I spelled.

I know why I keep thinking of this. It's because as Pat can sense, I am getting into serious trouble with my increasing embodiment.

I get so sick of a liquid diet going directly to my intestines. My lost body used to have food. Eating was ecstasy. I want my body back!

Sleepless

I have been moved to the Veteran's Hospital, and I have been fighting to obtain full control of my computer in my hospital room. The basic problem is that people haven't been able to handle the fact that my mind is not sleeping. Actually no one's mind sleeps. It is the body which sleeps. The body needs sleep times undisturbed by mind. In fact, our bodies are paralyzed when we sleep just as my body is permanently paralyzed now. Our bodies are insulated from the mind by this paralysis because our minds keep going during sleep. We call it dreaming when we become aware of it. One way of describing my present mental state is that I have gained 24 hour self-conscious control of my mind cut off from my lost and paralyzed body. This condition is known to science and is called "lucid dreaming." People all over the world are reading books that I've written about sleep and dreaming, yet the hospital won't believe me, the expert, when I say that I'm awake all night. They take my computer away every night so that no one will steal it (they say) while I'm asleep. Then Susy has a hassle every morning getting it back. She solved that by taking it home every night herself, and then bringing it back in her little wheeled shopping cart in the morning.

In the meantime they have apparently decided that the physical therapy I've been getting isn't going anywhere. The doctors can't do anything more. I'm neither dead nor alive according to the hospital bureaucracy. I'm forever fighting them. They view my departure with relief. I view my departure with relief. Everyone wins.

The tragedy is mine. It may be that my mind's movement back

into my imagined body has gone as far as it will go. My embodiment may be limited to my computer. With an electronic command hook up at home I could use the phone, lock and unlock the front door for visitors, turn the lights off and on, adjust the temperature, moving my mind through my house even though my body is lying in bed immobilized. Through my computer, I can make the whole house my body. Through the computer internet I can make the world my body. Yet I cannot give up the thought of trying to get back into my own body. They all thought that my body was going to die. They all thought my mind was dead. I've beaten them before. Can I do it again? I can! First, I'm going to get out of this hospital.

·

Isis

I'm through with the dead hospital room and the bureaucracy. They have brought me to my home. They wheeled me into the house through the front door, and they couldn't get me through the clutter of things. I'd forgotten how huge this house is – and how cluttered with things. I was left looking at the ceiling of the living room while they reconnoitered. Everything, the pictures, the grandfather clock, the big mantle piece all seemed to be leaning over me. These were parts of my life. After the cold sterility of the hospital room, which had not made much impression on me, I was seeing for the first time. And my house was seeing me back. My eyes were having a rich warm feast of these physical garments of my life. My house held me and said, "Hello lover."

People have always said that our house was so cluttered with "things" that we couldn't walk through it. They were right. I love it more than ever. It's myself! Let me drown in things.

They had to wheel me back out and in again through the french doors into the library – my favorite room. There was my statue of Kuan Li, the Goddess of Mercy, gleaming in soft gold in her niche. Further along was the almost life-sized Virgin Mary, Our Lady of Fatima, shining pure white with a blue cape. I gave it to Susy many years ago, after I had picked it up coming back from lecturing in Italy.

I was hoisted onto a hospital-type bed right under the Virgin Mary. What a great idea Susy must have had, putting me right here where the Virgin can constantly bless me. The rows of books, my dear old friends, let their good will descend upon me as a benediction.

This room looks out over the gardens and pool. It's full of light. I stay here all the time because it's so hard to move me. But this is all I need. Susy has a narrow bed right beside mine. Here we are in our house. Here among all these material things is where I will be reunited with my material body.

My greatest disappointment was Isis, my German Shepherd dog. We had always been inseparable when I was at home. She came in that first day, looked at me, sniffed my body, whined, looked confused and then slunk outside. She spent the rest of the day howling out there. She obviously recognized my body, but there was something wrong. Did she sense that my spirit wasn't there? Was it like someone seeing a ghost? It makes me think of the decorticated cat experiment Bill, Pat and I were involved with years ago. Only now I am the decorticated cat and Isis won't admit I exist. Isis, I suppose you only can know me when I'm connected to my body. My body must seem like meat to you if my mind is not in control of it – very confusing. There is no way you can sense my disembodied mind indirectly, like Bill and Pat.

Isis hasn't been willing to come back into the house since. Perhaps it is a haunted house to her now. I miss her. I'd been looking forward so to seeing her. I hate to admit this, but Isis is really getting to me. Susy says she paces back and forth outside the library all day. At night when everything is still I can hear her long ululating howl of pure despair. Does she know something that I'm not able to admit to myself?

I Just Want To be Safe and Loved

An old friend of Susy's, Vangy, a doctor's wife, comes in and they go into the next room for a talk. Still I can hear everything they say. Vangy has tinted red hair and numerous face lifts. She is soignee with a well-preserved figure. She's not exactly Susy's type. As usual they talk as people do as though I weren't there. It's obvious Vangy thinks I'm dead – just a dead body, artificially kept in a semi-living state. Susy has been telling Vangy about the day and about how tired and discouraged she feels. Life has become pretty flat for her.

Vangy says, "Listen, sweetheart, having to deal with these three old men, two of them doddering and the other, your man, dying or worse, has got to be discouraging. I know Patton is in his seventies, Bill is in his sixties, and well, James was about to turn sixty, wasn't he? I know those old rascals. And then all three of them do consulting without ever letting you into their minds – and answering questions with questions. How can you stand all that? You've put up with a lot! James was the glamorous one, so sleek and sophisticated. His patients were the beautiful people. He was so admired. You've lived a technicolor life. You're used to it. I suppose everything has turned black and white now."

Susy falters, "I didn't want glamorous. I like black and white. I just wanted to be safe and loved. I had never ever thought of James becoming so important all over the world."

Vangy continues, "Susy, you know James is gone. What are these two friends of his doing for him? They're just talking. They can't give him a body. You'd better face up to it. He's always going to be paralyzed."

Susy got up and gave herself a shake, "Enough. That's what Pat believes, that he will always be paralyzed. I fought Pat about that, but really I'm ready to take James however he is."

Communication

I've been overwhelmed with my new ability to express my thinking directly into words. Words are so much easier, more precise, and so much more fun. I don't even want to think about that desperate time when I fought just to keep my mind from dissolving. I have been looking forward eagerly to Pat's arrival.

He ambles in festooned with wires and boxes. He puts a finger to his lips, comes over and unplugs the big lamp between my bed and Susy's. The lamp had been on, and now this part of the room is plunged into shadow. The Virgin Mary seems to retreat. He plugs the lamp into a small box with a little antenna on top. Then I can hear him plug the box into the wall socket as he drops out of the range of my sight. The lamp comes back on. The Virgin Mary seems to lean back over me. What is this all about?

He picks up a hula hoop he has brought in with him and goes around to the other side of my bed. Standing like a stage magician, he displays the hoop and puts it over his head. It slips down around his body to the floor. Is this meant to signify that there are no wires? O.K. No wires. He steps out of it, sits in a chair, and stares at me solemnly. His eyelids always droop at the outside corners. Now they begin to droop a little more. His face seems to grow soft and out of focus. Suddenly the lamp goes out. Then the lamp comes on I'm startled. This is all very irritating and a little sinister.

I swivel my eyes to Pat. He smiles, his first expression since coming in. He looks at the lamp. It goes out. Then it quickly comes back on. After a moment, off and quickly back on — then off and quickly back on a third time. The next time the lamp goes off, it stays off for a longer time and repeats that three times. Then it goes quickly off and on again three times. Short, short, short – long, long, long – short, short, short. S O S. It's Morse Code from the lamp! Of course....

The son of a bitch. If I could move I would kill him. As my eyes turn towards him, he reaches into his long white hair and delicately shows me a fine wire disappearing into his scalp. He has wired up some of his brain cells directly into an EEG converter which broadcasts a signal to my lamp. I'll bet he has been practicing controlling his brain wave frequencies so he could send me Morse code. The rat, frightening me like that.

I look at my computer control board. *Up yours. Cheap parlor trick.*

My lamp starts flashing again. I am irritated; still I can't resist following and decoding the flashes. I had, after all, learned Morse code in the army. Pat's body seems to have become inert, slacked back in his chair. Only his greenish-brown eyes glint through his lashes.

The lamp flashes a long message. Had to do this before talking. Brain waves controlled by disconnecting mind from body. When talk vocally become embodied again.

I notice I am looking at the lamp instead of Pat. I don't have to. The flashes fill the room as though the message was in the air. As it is actually. One of the things that used to really irritate me was when Pat's eyes would drift around the room as though my message was coming from the air instead of from me – from my body. Now I am doing the same thing.

Then it suddenly strikes me. I am realizing that this is indeed a mental communication. Pat's mind is momentarily disconnected from most of his brain, as my mind seems to be permanently disconnected from most of my brain. Of course his disconnection is much less complete than mine, and he had the choice, curse him.

But his point is, I suppose, that if we both have disembodied minds, the quality of our communication will be enhanced; we will be approaching a different dimension. He has made his point dramatically. I am convinced.

Also, I realized, he was making a point about the relation of brain cells to subjective mental functioning. He had edited one of Barbara Brown's books. She was the scientist who had conceived of biofeedback in the 60s. Pat had been involved in biofeedback research and had a hand in developing some electronic equipment for brain wave experiments contrasting the two sides of the brain.

I looked at my computer and sent him this message using my mechanical voice. The computer's voice is so inhuman that it's hard to understand. Pat hates it. I love it when it irritates him. *Are you implying that if you could send a complex message using only a few brain cells, why couldn't a self-conscious, subjective mind function with only a few brain cells?*

The lamp flashed, Yes.

From a research point of view there are holes in that theory you could drive a truck through, but it's an intriguing possibility that my existence tends to validate. Are you implying that I could get along with even fewer brain cells than I now have left?

A Yes flashed in the air of the room.

I send back, *Forget it. Leave my brain cells alone. I'm going for gourmet dinners and good sex. I've got the bit in my teeth, and I'm on my way. You've made your point, and I agree with it. I've spent my life thinking, teaching and writing about mind, but I'm not your experiment anymore.*

The lamp started to flash and then stopped. Pat let out a long sigh, shook himself and sat up. He opened his mouth and started to talk.

"I've been going around with my eyes almost closed and with ear plugs to protect myself from this disgusting physical environment you're so obsessed with, you sensual libertine."

After Pat finally started talking, he couldn't stop. You could see he had been missing his physical existence. He got out of the chair and started pacing around.

Pat wanted to hook me up more or less permanently to a little EEG receiver he had brought for me.

"Look," he said, "what if no one puts your computer in front of your face? You can't communicate. With this you can communicate using just what's inside your head. It's like opening your garage door by pushing the button on your remote control. Only instead of pushing a button, you activate a few brain cells inside your head."

He adds, "I could fix this so you could control the lights all over the house. It wouldn't matter where other people were; you could still contact them. If you got bored in the middle of the night, you could turn the lights on and off and communicate with the neighbors too. The meditative technique to enable you to do this isn't so esoteric. You would need to practice a bit, that's all."

I let him hook me up a few days later, but I'm not motivated to use it. I'm focusing on getting back into my body. I know what he wants. He's trying to see if we can communicate directly mind to mind – more experimenting. But I'm tired of being a guinea pig.

Suzy's View

Susy is standing before me, her feet spread apart – implacable. "It's all so simple for you. Everyone knows how great and famous you are. Everyone doesn't know how hard it is on me. Well, where is everyone? They're not here. They don't have any idea of the way I'm taken advantage of. I've let you take advantage of me ever since I was sixteen years old in high school. Here I am at the end of my life, and you're still doing it. What's been the matter with me all my life?"

She continues, "At the hospital in Akron I said, 'You can have him; I don't want him.' My divorce proceedings were on the way. I could have been free of you and starting to make a life of my own. Listen to that – the unthinkable, a life of my own. But how could I leave your motionless body in a far-off city? Maybe I thought you would soon be dead, and I'd be free at last."

She then says, "I am just about ready to quit. Not only do I have to take care of your body and the house and all your activities. I have to move your body here and there. Bill has helped in the moving some, but now he's in a situation where he can't do it anymore. You had better pay attention to what I'm saying. I'm exhausted, and I have no life of my own."

I know Susy has not had a life of her own since marrying me. We don't have much money now, and I get her to buy me books and things, and then its gone. No more money for her to spend. Actually Susy is in charge of her life now for the first time since we've been married. She is in control of what I spend and whom I see. She controls what happens around me. She can pull the plug on my computer any time she feels like it. I am absolutely at her mercy. At last she is in complete control.

Think of it Susy, I say. *This is too good an opportunity to throw away by just walking out. Think of the power you have at last. Live it up!*

Will Susy be able to overcome all those years of being dominated by my position and professional power? Our love story has been both exciting and tragic. We still love each other.

Susy dropped in a chair and said to me. "How nice it is that everyone is living such a beautiful exciting life leaving me to take care of a two-hundred pound baby. People are so entranced with your mind that they forget your body. It is unresponsive and inert. At the same time all of its bodily functions are going on automatically. Your body is in diapers, and it regularly produces bowel movements like a two-hundred pound body does. Sometimes the diaper can't contain it all. And then there's the diarrhea. I have to contend with all this every single day. The daily pile of sheets and soiled pajamas. The smell seems to linger in my nostrils day and night. Also you drool like a baby, but a lot more than a baby could produce."

She goes on, "Why am I here constantly wiping your face, why don't I let you drool? But I can't. You are my baby. I am beginning to realize that I have been looking after you all our lives together. You have always been so heedless and helpless. You never looked after me."

She sighs, "I was thinking back to our marriage. I was so young. I thought I would have someone to watch over me and protect me – and cherish me."

It is late afternoon. I know that the sink is full of dishes and no vacuuming has been done. Dirty sheets and my dirty diapers are piled by the washing machine. But Susy was not attending to any of those necessities. Her slight figure was in the bedroom trying to get me dressed properly for the evening. She has recently turned sixty-four and her arthritis was particularly painful that day. And she was trying to turn a two-hundred pound paralyzed body on its side to get a paralyzed arm into a shirt sleeve.

She sighs and stops for a moment I can see her frustration. How could she possibly keep going? Also there is the anger at me because I had ordered eighty-eight dollars worth of new books on my computer, and she could have used that money to get some household help. I've never had any sense of money.

Susy has me dressed finally and is maneuvering my body into the hydraulic lift that moved it out of the bed and into the wheelchair. Handling my body was like handling a two-hundred pound sack of wheat. It is hard to hold and maneuver. Any little imbalance and this body sagged over the restraints. It is so hard to get back into position again. She pumps the hydraulic lift with a hand lever, getting me into the air and into the wheelchair. People see my body finally situated in the chair and think I am sitting there. I'm not. My body is held in place by gravity.

Susy rolled me down the hall and maneuvered me out to the driveway. Our van has a wheelchair lift. That has to be adjusted just right. The whole thing collapsed under my weight once and scared her to death. It also cost four thousand dollars we didn't have to get fixed.

I often look at my condition objectively. My conclusion is that I am not much good to anybody. I may be of some emotional value to Susy, but that is balanced out by the stress and pain that I cause her.

This kind of life is ridiculous. Susy can't keep it up. Why can't I at least thank her for what she does? For some reason it seems I would rather die than thank her.

Depression

I find myself bogged down with trying to get my body back. Maybe there is a lesson in all this. Once more I've thought I could have it all. Wrong again! I give up; it is too much for me to figure out. Why am I thinking of John Parrish, my freshman English teacher who ultimately drowned himself when he learned he had cancer? Maybe he tried to figure it out, too, but gave up and concluded that life wasn't worth it.

Would I have the courage to kill myself? Do I have the ability to, anyway? I must be awfully depressed.

Bill came in. "How are you?"

Depressed, I answered.

"Why?"

General circumstances.

"But remember that you are in many ways a unique medical and psychological case."

Of course Bill had to bring that up. My computer wrote, *I have a strong tendency to identify with my previous life, and to deny the stroke. My present life is, of course, a new way of life. I am a pair of eyes and a pair of ears connected to a portion of my brain. I can't eat or drink or taste or smell. I can't feel that I have a body. A mental life of thinking, imagination and spiritual interaction with others should be plenty. I find that I haven't adjusted to it fully.*

"Find a purpose," said Bill, reading what I had written.

That's the hardest part, I think of Rollo May and the thesis, in one of his books, that mankind will go to almost any length to avoid realizing his — or her — true freedom.

Bill answers, "I think the book was *Escape from Freedom.* Yes, freedom is scary."

It is also a terrible responsibility to think that we might be co-creators of our world. This concern with freedom fascinates me since from one point of view I have no freedom – I cannot perform any body function, although I sometimes try. From another point of view I have complete freedom since there is nothing physical that I have to do. It's odd being a mind without being able to affect anything.

Bill laughs and goes off to attend to his patients. Susy props me up – which is no easy matter. Then I write for several hours, which is laborious. Then I read for several hours until the night-time TV shows start. My purpose is to stay distracted for as long as possible and hope that those awful times when only I am awake will pass without my mind unravelling. That would be a usual day, a successful day.

Every night I lie awake. It's at those times that I am most likely to think about my condition and to feel depressed. The years of sameness stretch out before me like a seemingly endless line of telephone poles along the highway. What am I to do? Already the array of TV shows seems meaningless. Yes, I can still read, but what? There is simply no way to apply anything that I might learn. It is difficult to motivate myself with just improving myself, art for arts sake as it were. That's what not having a body has robbed me of – the ability to contact the world directly.

Wait a minute, isn't that really the condition of all of us all the time? Yes it is! Of course it is. We simply learn to ignore the time it takes for nerve impulses to travel up and down the spinal cord. Technically speaking we are all living a split second behind the instant of immediate reality. I am living in an immediate mental reality.

If I allow myself to think while lying awake I soon try to figure a way out of my difficulties when they are actually opportunities. No wonder I'm depressed! The hopelessness of my situation can hit me at any time, no matter what I am doing, if I do not keep my mind occupied. I have been through the sequence many times. There is one logical action I could take – suicide. But I don't see how I could pull it off. I am even helpless in that, the final solution. I could not even kill myself without someone helping me.

I often think that everyone would be better off without me. Caring for me is a burden for Susy. It leaves little room for anything else. If I could have regained my body, my appetite, my sexual activities – but that is clearly not possible now. The medical approach to giving me my body has failed. Only I can know the burden of thinking twenty-four hours a day or dying. As I age I am sure to become a problem for my children, especially if Susy predeceases me. They would have to care for me or put me into a nursing home. A nursing home seems like endless boredom to me, particularly if my time at the hospital is characteristic of life in an institution.

If I could really talk I could probably stay interested in my companions, since people are intrinsically interesting. But since I can't, I am closeted more than I want to be with my own thoughts. Would it be better for everyone if I were dead?

I no longer fit into the social fabric of the society and have become a net debit rather than an asset.

In a practical sense, I did die at the time of the stroke. Everything since has been a pale life after death, a state in which my lost body has been kept alive by heroic measures, by the tracheotomy and things like that. Perhaps I was "meant" to die at the time of the stroke. This strange half-life was the result. It gave me more life to be sure, but what a piece of a life!

Would you rather be dead, I ask myself? No, while there is life there is still hope, hope that the big puzzle can be solved, hope that meaning can finally be found. It probably won't be found, and I will finally die just as confused as I ever was, but there is hope that it can be different.

The trouble is that we expect life to imitate art. We expect there to be some purpose to make sense of it all. The possibility that there is no purpose becomes almost unthinkable, so we invent one. We imagine a last judgement whose outcome is supremely important. It would be ironic if the last judgement turned out to be a self-judgement, as if God turned to you and asked, "Well what do you think – was it all worthwhile or not?"

I've thought about suicide, God but I don't have the guts or the strength, either. Someone would have to help me, and that's not fair to the other person. At worst it makes them an accessory in murder. But if there were someone around like that "Dr. Death" on TV – I think his name was Kervorkian – I would be tempted to commit suicide. This is a morbid conversation! I'm sorry.

The first decision with Dr. Herrer was too quick. There was no time to reflect. There was no time to consider the imposition on others, on Susy. Right now I'm not so sure living was the right choice, but I would prefer that death be painless. We treat animals better than people – putting them to sleep painlessly.

What do I have to look forward to?

There's always writing – I guess I still care about that. One reason I did not seriously think of suicide was that I could think of no way to do it. An overdose of medication was not possible. I did not have a gun. Besides, I would have to persuade someone to bring it and use it. I even thought of starving myself, but the food just goes down the tube to my body's intestines. They could feed me through that even if I chose not to eat. I'm disconnected. It has nothing to do with me. It seems I was meant to live out my normal lifespan. But can I endure years of a meaningless existence?

The book that Pat and I are working on has some meaning. Is it enough? For the time being, yes. At least, it will have to do. But Pat estimates that it is two-thirds finished. What then? Hold on buddy, I tell myself. One day at a time, one day at a time. The evil of the day is sufficient thereto.

Suicide

I have no reason to live other than an irrational fear of dying – not of death, which is inevitable, but of the process itself. I have reached the obvious conclusion.

The next time Bill comes I try to bring up the subject. I need help.

Bill, I need some help.

"With what, old buddy?"

He tapped his mechanical pencil. After a long pause he said simply, "I wouldn't."

l was looking at the pattern of the plaster on the ceiling, but my mind was on other things. The sheer particularity of the world seemed somehow beautiful, and the thoughts of leaving it voluntarily seemed somehow based on abstractions.

Bill continued, "I won't help you kill yourself, if that's what you're asking. Maybe you could learn something from your condition – for example, is it worth living a pure life of the mind? You're like a natural experiment. I'd suggest you see it through!" this was said with his usual quiet voice. A casual observer might think we were talking about nothing more important than the price of potatoes.

I often think of Pat at such times. He always seems so laid-back. I attribute it to his attitude toward life. Everything seems interesting to him, but nothing seems too important. I wish I had more of the same attitude.

People have become more important to me now. I suppose it is because I can no longer discount their motives. Since I no longer have anything to offer anyone, they must be interested just because they care. Susy is the best example of this.

The book Patton and I have decided to write would be an important contribution. We've gotten back together in faith and affection after our big argument. That's good, but he is not here now.

There is not the possibility of much of anything – except reading. But what to read? From before my stroke, I had enough unread books on hand to last several years. My reading time, several hours each day, was about evenly divided among books on psychological research, books on philosophy and religion, and books of general cultural interest, such as books on history.

Sometimes while reading I forget myself for a few moments. I am momentarily lost in the author's prose. It is a lot like hypnosis. At some level you know you are doing something – reading or "being hypnotized" – but at moments you forget and then the stimulus takes on the trappings of reality, much as in a dream. Would that I could induce it every time I wanted to! I would probably spend my life in a dream state. It seems much preferable to the hard reality. Still in my fantasies I can walk and talk, just like normal men.

Sex is an interesting topic, particularly when separated from the body, as I am. I still have sexual thoughts, lots of them. But that's it – they're just thoughts, not impulses to action. I have the thought and it's disconnected from any impulse to act on it, sort of purely aesthetic. I look at women as pure works of art, to be enjoyed but not touched. This is a new attitude, and I rather like it. My body makes no demands on my mind.

Sex is a funny appetite. It is satisfied, not like the regular appetite for food, by taking something into the body, but by the use for a while of another body. There seems little doubt that sex enters into all that we do. When talking to any woman, a man also thinks of her, at least in part of his mind, as a sexual partner. This goes on with dim awareness perhaps no matter what else is going on in the transaction. At least it always used to when my body was intact, before the stroke.

I tried to get across to Bill this change in perspective the next time he visited.

He didn't seem impressed and commented, "So your body was

only a vehicle for the illicit lusts of sex and the immoderate gluttony of food. Would you still be willing to sell your soul for sex and food?"

You bet! Especially food. In fact it was one of the few appetites that one could rely on being there day after day. Maybe we should give it more prominence because of its reliability. But when it's not possible, it's just another example of an embodied existence I don't have.

After Bill left, I endured another terrible bout of depression. I had reached out, sold my soul in a way, for the promise of re-embodiment – physical therapy. But the price was giving up, losing faith and actually betraying much of my disembodied mental facilities. Now I'm stuck.

I have to admit that when I had a body, I shuddered at the thought of dying from not being able to breathe enough, which is what would happen with an overdose. But, maybe the shudder was at death itself. I wasn't resigned to death. It was a case of the higher mind, the human part, overruling the natural animal instinct to die when body didn't work.

What, No Emotion?

I keep telling Bill I am depressed. What do I mean depressed? Depression is a low level of emotions. There has been no "affect" in my life. In that meaning of depression, I have been "depressed" ever since my stroke. I've got to think about this.

Depression. I talk the patient into releasing her body's emotions...*body's emotion.* Or I prescribe Prozac. In both cases it is *body's* emotion.

Relief: The patient talks until she feels relief – like a heavy weight lifted off her shoulders. But that is felt as *body* relaxation.

Wow! The patient can do that, but I can't. I cannot feel my body. For me relaxation means mental relaxation. Suicide was a mental load – not a bodily one. There must be another answer.

What.

I've had an astounding revelation. I have no emotions. Emotions are body's ways of thinking. When I've been thinking about suicide it's been a mental reality only, no emotion. My thoughts have been about what is the logical thing to do. I'm missing not only my body but my body's ways of thinking. I have none of my body's instincts. I have to realize that instinct is for the preservation of my body. It is a genetic product of evolution – of reacting to the environment. Without my body, my mind has no ups and downs of emotional affect.

Does this mean I am no longer human, that I am only a mental machine following cause and effect reasoning? Will people think of me as a non-human freak, with no heart, if they suspect that I have no emotional instincts. Heart. As a body sense, "heart" is associated with passion. But as mental reality, isn't also heart associated with compassion? Isn't compassion spiritual? If having no body makes me less than human, couldn't it also imply an opportunity to become more than human? Emotions tie humans to their animal instincts. Our bodies are animal bodies. Can my lack of emotions be not only a terrible loss but also an awesome opportunity? My mind is the reality of cultural development. My mind began where my body's evolution ended. My mental childhood development absorbed the reality of my thousands of years-old cultural evolution, that is reality – spiritual reality! I can do more, and I will.

The Madonna by my bed seems to be leaning over me with no pity at all. Purity can be very hard on those of us who are not so pure. Her pure ceramic face would crush me if she fell over. Why did I stop praying to you, Madonna? You were my girl, ready to give me love and take me to your beautiful bosom. Won't you take me away from all of this?

Yes, maybe she can! I've been so caught up in the failure of medicine to give me my body back, I've forgotten God and the spirit. The medical establishment knew I couldn't get my body back, but they couldn't stand my mind continuing to live. I'll be damned if I'll commit suicide just to make them feel better. I've been caught between the mental life of mental interactions with others and the physical life of physical interactions with others. But there is God and the spirit – and always has been. The oldest organized human thought was about how God and the spirit created humankind. God and the spirit are inseparable from human thought. My mental thought and its interaction with other humans needs interaction with God and the spirit – there is my salvation. I will not be a sick man. I will be a reborn man. If that is to be my way, I know what I must do. They will find out about it in my testament.

The Testament of James Hall

As will become apparent, I, Patton, have had to write this chapter of James' story. Bill telephoned me while I was in New York. "I'm worried about James," he said. "He's fallen into a deep depression. He's given up after investing so much hope and care into his physical recovery. He is not making any more progress in regaining control of his body. He can't get back to his earlier excitement about his disembodied mental freedom. He is trapped in a classic double bind with nowhere to go. I think he has even given up trying to seduce the Madonna by his bed."

I caught the next plane for home and drove straight to James' house from the airport. The lawn was overgrown. The house looked deserted.

A sad and subdued Susy let me in. The living room had changed its atmosphere from overcrowded to funereal. The air was dead, with dust clinging to every surface. The two mandalas on the wall had become round baleful eyes seeing doom.

Susy whispered, "He won't open his eyes. I feed him through the tube into his intestines and care for him, but I'm not even sure he knows I'm there."

She handed me some sheets of paper, "This was on the computer. I've printed it out."

These are the words he left. The papers were titled:

A Testament

I'm through with thoughts of suicide now. If they were, in fact thoughts of suicide, or were just selfish ways of drawing attention to myself. Pat was right. Thoughts of body make me selfish. Whatever, I'm through with all that. Now that I understand how I'm missing body emotions in my mental world, I understand how I got myself in a rational double bind.

My mental world as it exists, even with all the wonderful interactions I'm having with others, is not enough. I can't get body's emotions back. I can only think rationally. In the abstract, my greatest fear has been that if I ever stopped thinking rationally my mind would just dissolve into the universe and I would be lost. That may have been true in the beginning, but is it true now?

I propose to stop thinking rationally and put myself into the hands of God and the spirit. If I can't have body's emotions, perhaps I can have spiritual emotion, the universal love and compassion of God in my thoughts. And perhaps have rational thought where it's appropriate as well. But now I have to give up abstract thinking and put myself in the hands of God.

Do you think that someone like myself could be redeemed? I'm going to bet my life on finding redemption.

I appreciate all the time Pat and Bill have spent trying to establish communication with me. And I value our work together all these years. Please thank the directors of Western Human Sciences Institute for approving this computer.

I will just go as far as I can without losing the option of coming back. In case I shouldn't make it back, I want to leave you with a simple conviction I have acquired. I have become a being of pure consciousness and still live as myself – a human being. I am convinced that in the future there will be souls like me – beings with only tenuous connections to physical life. Does the word, "angel" describe humankind's age old understanding of soul? I have begun to sense something. If I get back, I will bring something beautiful.

Also, it is clear that if we are to have souls, we will have to create them. As Barbara Hannah said, "Mind constructs a unique immaterial space of its own." Over a lifetime mind can create a soul – that which is most vital to human beings. Doesn't soul mean simply what lives beyond body. If our minds are to live on beyond our bodies, it will be our doing. I think of sin now as being the willful dissolution of my mind. You have watched me flirt with it in moments of depression. The more I have centered on body self, the more selfish and depressed I have become. The more I have accepted being a mind disconnected from the body, the less selfish I have become. Selfishness creates depression and dissolution. So if I were to make a second point, it would be this.

Sin is the body. Think of definitions of sin. Aren't they about the body doing something? Scientific advances in the near future may create the possibility of living comfortably as minds with little body. Only minds transcending the body will be able to do that.

I don't want this read by others unless I come back. It could be so easily misinterpreted by anyone who was not aware of the unbelievable scientific adventures we've had since my mind was disconnected from my body by that stroke. I know the hospital records and the records at Western Human Sciences Institute are incontrovertible, but they have to be understood first. Mine is not a story about a physical tragedy but about the ability of mind to exist without body.

A Leap of Faith

Leaving the Testament with Susy, I made my way back through the silent rooms to the library. There was a feel of decay over everything. A floor board creaked under my weight and I jumped, heart pounding. I leaned my head against the library door, hands together, and meditated for a moment. I had to be totally receptive – without fear or defenses when I went in.

As I entered the library, shadows moved. The light from the setting sun is dim. Leaves from the garden shrubbery outside the windows hang limp and disconsolate, cut off from the water which gives them life.

The Madonna gleamed pale and tall by James' bed in the dim light. I could just see James' still form as I made my way across a clutter so forbidding it seemed malevolent.

This Virgin Mary, who has meant so much to James and has watched over him wore a golden crown. In this statue she was the Madonna of Fatima, worker of miracles in the midst of destruction. For the first time I realized there was a parallel between this Madonna and the Hindu Goddess Kali, who, with her multiple sets of arms, dances about both life and death.

As I crouched by James' bed the Madonna seemed to again lean over James threateningly. I placed a trembling hand over one of James' hands. There is no life there. Wait! There was a pulse. What was going on here? Then I remembered my early conversations with James about the stroke. The cold fingers of shock felt their way through me. In his testament that I had just put down, James had described his struggle to keep his mind from unraveling and dissolving into the universal mind. He had to deliberately discipline his thoughts into rational patterns and he interacted with those around him even when he couldn't communicate with them. That was how he had avoided becoming a vegetable. He was going to give up the rational abstract thinking which had kept his mind together and see if the mind of God was the reality.

"Damn you, James," I whispered, "You can't go off and leave this useless body here for us to look after. You know only too well what that's like."

I didn't know whether James was willfully refusing to communicate, or whether his mind was dissolving or whether his mind was tired of using the computer or whether he was tired of existing on the edge of embodiment and disembodiment. Or perhaps he had given his will up to "God's" will.

I couldn't let James go. The image of the gold-crowned Madonna rising so perilously over him filled my mind. I could pray to her. She was not painted statuary at all, but alive. I could feel the living limbs beneath the sheer blue robe. Her living breasts rose and fell. My God! Of course! James hasn't run out of women. There is still the virtual Madonna.

I remembered a lecture from long ago given by Marie Louise Von Franz. She had been Jung's pupil and James' mentor when he attended the Jung Institute in Zurich. She had written something once that came to my mind now.

At our peril we forget that the archetypical madonna is alive in the spirit, that she has spiritual flesh and living desires for the divine intimacy we sometimes mistake for sex.

James has always been a sucker for sex, but perhaps it was more for the divine intimacy than it was through physical sex. I now knew what to do. If anything will draw James out from the Universe, this was it. Sorry, Madonna. That's the way I see it, and that's the way I'll play it.

I spoke aloud in that silent room. The sound of my voice startled me. "James, the Madonna is right here by your bed. Her breath is the perfume of delight. Her flesh is warm and full of desire for you. She wants you. She is waiting for you right here."

The room stays silent, dead. Time is a lost dimension. James' mind may be unravelling, but surely he can still hear through this body if he wants to. I'm sending out a message designed to attract his attention. I am beginning to feel a little superstitious about using the Madonna as a hook for James' mind.

Suddenly, the light from the lamp by James' bed turned on. In that rude flash of light the real, heavy masonry of the statue of the Madonna appeared to be falling over to crush James in her embrace. I throw up my arm and shouted, "No!" Then the light turns off and she is back where she was. James' eyes are closed.

Then the light blinks again. I. Then three times. S. It's the Morse Code, damn him. He must be still hooked to the lamp.

I – S
S – H – E
R – E – A – L – L – Y
T – H – E – R – E
IS SHE REALLY THERE?
Then another message; I'M C O M I N G B A C K
Then, F R O M T H E U N I V E R S E
Then, I'M W A Y O U T
Then, V E I L S O F V I B R A T I O N S B E C O M I N G C O L O R S R E D B L U E Y E L L O W O V E R W H E L M I N G R U S H I N G T O O F A S T
After a long time, I F I M A K E I T I W I L L B R I N G S O M E T H I N G B E A U T I F U L

It might be that time didn't exist where he was. Everything may happen at once. Nothing had come through since that last message. Would he know the difference between a minute and a lifetime? I had no idea. James is the first adventurer of the disembodied universe.

I was convinced that James was coming back at any moment. Toward morning James' eyes opened, still glazed over with the beauty of eternity. There is no other sign, but I rushed around turning on lights. I also turned on James' eye-operated computer. This is it – human kinds' great moment. Someone is coming back from heaven, from God, from whatever was out there beyond the material world. I call Susy and Bill. This is more exciting than Columbus coming back from the New World. This is an adventurer coming back from the mental universe, from the wild unknown.

Locked In To Life

VII

The Wild Universe

A Beautiful Life

This is James back again. Pat apparently thought he was having some trouble getting me back, but I had no trouble. Pat exaggerates. I was coming back anyway, but I enjoyed using his little biofeedback trick on him. My brain cells, as few as there are now, were right here. But in truth I was spiritually far, far away. I open my eyes and see my computer. That was thoughtful of Pat, and there he is and Susy and Bill. They all look worried, but I'm at peace – no more fake depressions, no more fears about my mind dissolving. I'm working my computer now. It's a good feeling. OK, this is my adventure.

I've finally given up my body in a joyful release, and I'm bringing something beautiful to you all. I have had a transcendent vision of the reality of life. It isn't so very different from things we have thought about, – in fact – everything is beautiful. I will tell you about my adventures in the mental universe. You will need that as a foundation to appreciate the rest. Later I will tell you about the living beauty which it is my mission to bring back to you.

This mission has been revealed to me through my journey, I began to feel pregnant, filled up with a consciousness outside myself yet which was also my self. There was nothing physical, no body, only my thoughts. There was a rushing insistence, a tugging intention to whirl my thoughts away.

There had been no perception, only thought. As my thoughts sank down, there was a knowledge of the existence of gravity being focused into an impossibly hard point. I thought of being at the beginning of the universe. I began to be aware of vibration which became color. Suddenly everything was a hot red, so hot that it was yellow. I was whirled away into a relentless irresistible rushing. But my thoughts remained mine. The yellow picked up some streaks of cooler red. My thoughts were still yellow. Then my thoughts became red-streaked rushing yellow picked up green streaks, then blue and purple streaks. After the purple there was a bump, and all color was gone from my thoughts. My thoughts, myself, were transparent against the rushing colors around me. On occasion I still get a glimpse of that clarity.

How can I express the beauty of my universe?

Of course it is God's universe, but I find it is mine as well. I can begin by telling you how it has affected me. A remarkable change has colored my being. I have developed a sense of certainty in regard to things I had merely speculated about before. For example, in my vision the events of my life rushed around me. I now view each of them as an attempt to teach me something. Perhaps the most impressive change was in my feelings. I felt no aggression towards anyone. Rather I understood that I had been given time to be redeemed – for instance to examine every aspect of my intentions towards the three women who sued me for sexual misconduct. I no longer harbored aggressive thoughts about them. My life was a heaven and hell problem. The problem was to understand why I had thought and felt as I did. The experience colored my attitude about many things – God, Christianity, history, analytical psychology.

I felt as if I had been in the presence of some changing multi-personality that I called "god" in contrast to God as a single personal eternally unchanging being. In the rushing colors around me was a place of stillness surrounded by a clear membrane. I was below it, and above me was a shimmering statue. This "god" resembled the rushing colors of the universe held in place by the violent forces sweeping around it in ever-tightening orbits. This "god" was always changing. It was a center of multiple personal beings that couldn't exist without the rushing forces around it. The power of communication actually came from those forces.

The universe seemed big enough to hold all human thought in a never ending future. This place of rushing colors seemed available to any one who could still their abstract thinking and give themselves to the reality of "god."

The meaning of its message came to me in harmonic resonances. I believe that it has to do with the reality of compassion and honesty. It is clear that this message cannot exist in a static state but must be constantly revealed to me through the most precise examinations of my intentions throughout my life.

"God" seemed uninterested in what people thought but was exquisitely interested in why they thought it – what the intention, or the color, was. The intention was the mindscape of the thought.

Then I began examining all the events of my life as if they had been sent to me as lessons. This formula would be true for anyone. I am overwhelmed with awe at whatever intelligence could coordinate such a world of rushing veils – colors of thought.

I also grasped the intuitive truth that the life of pure consciousness is like disembodied breathing – the greater the mental contraction, the greater the mental expansion. This rhythm is as vital to the mind as breathing is to the body. I received a definite revelation that we exist in order to learn and that in this process of mental contracting and expanding, the death of the body is nothing. The rush of life I was experiencing didn't stop with bodily death and seemed a spiral evolutionary process always moving into the future. Its unfolding continued endlessly on different levels.

My ambivalent fear of losing my body had decreased. The body really did not matter. I realized that my orientation had subtly changed from a nostalgic yearning for my idealized physical childhood toward an expectation of what the future might bring in the wild mental universe.

A Crackling in the Air

I remember Pat saying that as I returned there was a crackling in the air as though powerful currents had swept through the room leaving things seeming clean and sparkling.

But the next meeting of my friends kept getting delayed. As though a beacon had suddenly been lit, people of all kinds began to visit even though there had been no attempt to communicate my return. Also these people were no longer put off by being in the presence of this "dead body." I would produce short sentences on my computer about pure self-intention and the art of self-intentioned interactions. I repeated one constant refrain: nothing mental is hidden from "god."

Susy seemed to sparkle in thought and in her physical appearance. The feel of the house brightened. The rooms seemed lighter and less cluttered. My room was especially bright. If you recall, it had been my old library with doors opening out to the garden and pool. The foliage that had seemed dry and dreary before now seemed brighter. Someone must have done some watering. Part of the bright feeling in the room seemed to be coming in from the outside. Isis, my dog, seemed somewhat happier and was content to approach at least as far as the door without getting upset over my body.

Psychotherapists began visiting for my interpretations of their client's dreams, and people who had been in psychotherapy themselves came to me seeking something. They did not know what it was except that it was not of this world. In cryptic ways, I gave them answers, solutions, and solace. Something strange began to happen. Some of the physicians who had been most upset by my disembodied mind began to drop by. Even Dr. Herrer, who had been so disturbed by my mental existence, came by after months of no contact at all. He found the same motionless body with the same incomprehensible means of producing written words with almost unnoticeable eye movements. However, I was not disturbed this time. He didn't seem to know how to speak to me or didn't feel there was anything he needed to say, yet was interested in my descriptions of colors and rushing veils of thought – as though it had struck some chord in Herrer's own experiences of life and death. Dr. Herrer has since helped liberate an electronic color feedback machine from the hospital for a few months. I find it useful in clarifying the qualities of color I found outside me in the universe. The colors were the spiritual vibrations and the limitless rush and flow of thoughts in the universe. There is a spiritual existence beyond us. Small groups are gathering around me, although I am disturbed by the presence of more than a few people at a time. I realized, the intimacy of one person to another is the only way to true being.

My body is strapped in a wheelchair. Visitors seem to be self-selected, mostly professionals, who feel a promise awaits them. These are some of the kinds of people who come: a scholar from India, a couple of young students from half-way around the world, a housewife, a catholic priest, a Zen master, a husband and wife who are both university professors, and a lawyer. They sit silently and at peace as my body is turned to receive them and my computer is arranged. The computer screen has been programmed to project letters large enough to be read by the group. They read some words about the body-self and the true mental self.

When questions are asked, I flash these words on my screen, *I have no information for you. Let us dance. Dance with our minds to the music of rushing mental colors. I will conduct the music through my computer.*

The Indian scholar becomes passionate about me as the hero who has journeyed beyond the world to bring back something new and precious. He mentions Prometheus who brought fire to human kind.

I flash the computer again, *Why did he bring fire? Why was he a hero?*

The lawyer feels we are all heroes to the extent we have compassion for the diverse and disadvantaged.

The housewife is outraged at "an attempt to bring politics into matters of the spirit."

I ask, *What is the why of compassion? What is political intention? How is it different from spirit?*

The Catholic priest smiles and suggests that Jesus has appeared in some strange forms – sometimes as a hero. He suggests that perhaps my 'god' who was present upon a higher plane or membrane might well have been the figure of Jesus. He mentions that this figure apparently sent my soul or "ghost" back as a hero to engage the physical world for many more years.

My computer screen, *Actually it was a large crouching male figure against a vaporous background, and we communicated without speaking. I did not connect it to Jesus.*

The Indian scholar finally proclaimed, "This is a chance for every person to be a hero for humankind by behaving with pure, good intentions."

The World Outside

On top of all this, The New York Times became aware of my story and sent a reporter down to Dallas to interview me. The reporter was a lovely lady named Dee Wedermeyer who spent several days with me. I invited her to one of my impromptu meetings.

There were twelve men and women there. A writer started things off by presenting his dream. He was climbing a ladder to see some kitchen cabinets. At the top he found a bag of cat food surrounded by mouse droppings. He pulled the cat food toward himself.

My computer encouraged the group to find associations. The writer saw cats as feminine and relaxed. Mice as pests. The dingy cabinets he associated with his life style.

My computer asked, *What does climb the ladder mean?*

"Advancing, reaching a goal or accomplishment," the writer said.

My computer, *What do you learn by changing perspective?*

"I learned something was there, something I've got to clean up," the writer said.

The group was now catching on, mice became symbols, mice in nursery rhymes and mice in mythology. Something seemed out of balance. The mouse and the cat were not there. Would that be in balance?

"My main relationship is out of balance, work is out of balance," the writer replies.

My computer, *If you became more catlike how would you change?*

"Smarter," the writer says.

More independent?

"Yeah, I think in a sense, my mood, whatever I'm thinking is dramatically affected by the way my wife is feeling toward me."

A woman in the group danced like a cat. She was a lazy cat, she stretched and arched her back. Another woman danced like a cat. She poked her nose in the air. Then the writer danced like a cat. He stretched out on the floor, smiling contentedly as if he would be happy to have his back scratched.

"Playful, comfortable," the writer said.

Dee seemed to get something out of the meeting and used it in her article for The New York Times.

The Little "I"

At last Patton and I arranged to be alone to try to consider the abstract scientific issues raised by my journey into a wild mental universe.

My computer screen, *I will only interact with individuals about specific personal issues, whether in a group or alone, and I will only use the computer to write about individual personal events – and only in terms of individual compassionate intentions. Compassion for me is a personal state of being.*

"Listen," says Pat, "I have to find some way of making sense of all this, some way of collating these individual encounters where you say cryptic things to individual people which enlighten them personally but no one else. I understand that there are no set rules to follow or even any systematic approach for people's longings to go beyond. I agree, but I need to have some true way of expressing a direction at the very least. You've given us some ways of being compassionate, but..."

I decided to give Pat more of a usable program.

It is being compassionate enough. Here goes. This is the point. I've got some years to redeem myself. That's it. I haven't been given any special instructions about what to do, but I know that I must redeem myself or perish. Also I know that to redeem myself, others connected to me will have to redeem themselves. But I have no control over what someone else does. I have no rules for salvation. I don't know of anything I or anyone else must do.

The only path I have been given to follow is to pay very close attention to why I do things. That means I must go back and examine my conscious intentions in the past. I see my consciousness as an uninterrupted flow from birth. I can't know the whys of my present unless I know the whys of my past. The process of examining my intentions can only apply to me. I can't tell you how to examine your intentions. In my vision of 'god' each of us is forever unique. Since we each exist only in relation to each other, I suspect we will discover our whys and our redemptions in relation to each other.

A personal growing intention to be true is reflected in the colors of pure consciousness. Remember that the universe is made of vibrations and each vibration is a color. You must hear the music of the colors of all the personal thoughts that are happening there. They are each unique events of a universal melody that in its rushing sweep is made up of each unique personal intention at each moment.

Perhaps I can suggest a central symbol. You know I am in the process of learning just as you are. I have not been given an ultimate revelation, but the thinking tone I have been getting is of the Tao, the Chinese understanding of life as a water-course always rushing but always being changed in direction by each and every personal intention that is compassionate enough in its place and time to be a living part of this 'divine' rushing. Tao saw it as water running down a mountain side that swerves and turns to account for every pebble and every blade of grass.

Only I see this rushing as not down as the Tao does, but out and up over the body of life – in a sexual way, and this is most important – the rushing has a sense of personality which the Tao doesn't.

I am trying to describe myself in the lower case but in quotes so as to be 'personal.' I am trying to get this dammed computer to designate my self, as I know I must, with a little 'i.' However, when I direct my mind to the space-bar symbol, the computer automatically capitalizes lower case i's. The little 'i' symbol is important in expressing the opening of my self to others and them to me so that we live in each other, and we speak for each other each with a little 'i.'

Using 'i' signifies the paradox that we are each unique and that we are also multi-personal relationships constantly changing.

Pat is stretched out in the leather easy chair. He jumps up, "That's it! We have been learning to communicate with each other beyond our alienating bodies. We are living in our minds rather than our bodies and we are all little 'i's.' That is the common symbol I was looking for—the little 'i.' It isn't the word it is the thought of 'i.' You can't abstract a little 'i.' Each little 'i' is changing and is unique. You want us all to be little 'i's.'"

Pat continues, "The concept of Tao is that changes by pebbles and blades of grass changes our lives. Your concept of Tao is that our little 'i's' become part of the sweep of colors which interacting together change our lives. The little 'i's' become our souls. When we die they continue to live, and change. These changes become rocks and pebbles of Taoism. It is all these little 'i's' in the universe that made up 'God.'"

Pat says, "I am not going to succumb to being in awe of you, James, but it's hard not to. What you're dredging up out of the universe is so exciting, exhilarating and inspiring. One thing is becoming clear to me as I experience the encounters going on here – I am a child of the universe, not of this planet. The planet is a great womb, but we are on the point of being born into the universe. That is our human heritage."

Then Pat leaves, going his own way with courage and resolve. *God bless him.*

The Green Man

Pat comes back the next day, "I see that the movement of your eyes on your computer has become so fast that I wonder if you are really using your eyes or just compelling the computer directly with your mind."

My computer prints, *Ah, who knows. Maybe a little of both.* (That will get him thinking.) *It would be better to direct such questions to me, the computer. After all I am James' body now.*

I will tell you as an illustration an Islamic story that you may remember about Khadir. He is a nature spirit, but is simultaneously a human being. Being physically alive gives him a color of nature. He is a green man. He meets Moses – the biblical Moses although this story is not in the Bible. They meet on the road and Khadir says, 'You may walk along with me if you wish, but you may not question what I do.'

Moses walks along the dusty track with him as it winds through the parched countryside. They encounter a beautiful young man bursting with life and health. Khadir promptly kills him and leaves his dead body sprawled by the side of the road. Khadir casually walks on. Moses is appalled. He bends over the young man and sees that he is dead.

Moses rushes after Khadir. 'You just killed him without even talking to him or asking his name. You murdered him! God will strike you down because you have violated one of his commandments.'

Khadir continues walking and without looking at Moses says, 'I am not subject to the rules of your God. I am liable only for my intentions. I told you not to question me. My thoughts are without boundaries. Body thinking needs explanations. Thought unbound from the body needs only intentions. The boy intended to murder his parents for their money. I am uninterested in the question of their money, but their compassionate love for each other is a beacon for the wild heaven that is the place you seek.'

Khadir's voice becomes faint as he walks away and disappears into the distance.

Pat replied, "If this is a story about true compassionate intention, then it is tough compassion. OK. But what if the murdered young man would have found compassion at the last moment and not killed his parents?"

He adds, "Let's go back; you say compassion is opening yourself up without conditions to another's personal compassionate intention. There are no rules for what that intention might be, but in this Khadir story, the existence of the parent's compassion versus the intention of the son to kill them is enough for Khadir to choose to murder the son. That is tough indeed."

I respond, *Khadir could have made a mistake in his intentions and would have been irrevocably damned. Killing someone is not the sin. The intention is the sin. Is it a compassionate intention? If your intention is wrong and you act on it, then you are irrevocably wrong.*

This is good, Pat is riled up now and pacing the floor.

My computer screen says, *If your child needs a stone but asks for bread, would you give him a stone or bread? Your intention must be for the compassion to give him a stone even if he thinks he needs bread. Intentions must be tough. The most you can do in this life is to always be compassionate to the best of your ability, and pray that you are not wrong. You could be betting your life. But you must choose. For example, consider Oedipus: He chose to kill his unknown father to protect himself and chose to marry his unknown mother in the process of getting a kingdom. He bet his life, and he was wrong. The Oedipus story is one of the most significant in humanity's inheritance. It uncouples what may happen from any knowable rational reasons.*

Pat says, "Right. We have talked about how no one has a privileged point of view. In any moment how can you locate your point of reference – is it to your self, to your dog, or the plane overhead? It's like Job's story in the Bible. From Job's point of view there was no rational reason for all the bad things that happened to him. That can be true for any of us. No matter how truly compassionate our intention may be, bad things may happen that are beyond our control. They may not have anything to do with us. An intention may never be achieved, but it can be attempted.

We can never know to what extent our intention has been fulfilled, but we must intend compassion as best we can."

The computer screen flashes, *Examining one's intentions is the ultimate art. There are no rules. The only condition is that the examination be honest and true to the best of our abilities. We can only be redeemed by constantly examining the events of our lives. An intention is a complex web of relations with other minds and with 'god's' wild rush of spirit.*

Pat shifts irritably in his chair, "But if we only care about saving our mental being – won't that create havoc on Earth? People will act any way they please and justify it by saying that it fulfills a higher mental goal. As in your example with Khadir, murder would be acceptable. Some people might evolve into more compassionate people and reach your vision of beauty, but many others might not."

Pat then says, "Remember the old saying that the road to hell is paved with good intentions. That saying emphasizes the importance of rules of behavior. You infer the opposite, that what counts is the intention. You seem to be taking away the rules altogether. In that case, we have lost any common way of interpreting human intentions. Can we be trusted to examine our good intentions without being tempted to justify our actions? Our psychological theories of human behavior are so over-determined, there are so many ways of explaining why we do what we do, that there is a great danger that people would make rules for examining their intentions. Such rules could then justify doing bad things to others."

I interrupt Pat. *My point is that there are no good intentions, only compassionate intentions, so there can be no justification for saying, 'I did a bad thing but my intentions were good.' Compassion breaks through and goes beyond morals and dogmas to pure intention. In his compassion for the prostitute Jesus asked who would cast the first stone. I am expressing an available direction for all of us everywhere to follow as we examine our lives without the need to justify them. As you know I have always been opposed to reducing psychotherapy to rules of behavior. That is also the basis of my opposition to rules of religion and other group rituals. They imprison the mind rather than freeing it to explore existence. Yes, I have always feared the possibility of substituting a new set of rules for the old ones. You are demonstrating how we can insure that this doesn't happen.*

Pat said, "Perhaps we could think of this in terms of spiritual evolution. In the past, one tried to align one's thinking with God's thinking by following mental rules. Now you are suggesting a radical change in mental evolution living in intimate daily contact with 'god' in order to save our mental being."

Now you are beginning to work it out for yourself.

Pat's eyes are sparkling, "Think of the freedom available to all who reach for it – freedom to live every hour of every day without defending or judging – yet lovingly examining the beauty to be found in life. It is the new mental art for everyone. We are all equal before 'god.' At last I know what that means. It means we are all equally able to reach out to 'god,' free to educate ourselves, free to work together on this green earth, free to live in our wild universe!"

I feel good. Pat must wait and live, and be conscious of each personal intention. He must interact with me more in particular moments of discovery and give up his abstractions. I am now spending more time on the book he and I are writing. It will introduce the public to my mental world. It will be a prophecy of how "people of the mind" can embark on a great adventure beyond all known boundaries of physical being.

I leave Pat with this line, *We live on the left hand of 'god' in faith and trust.*

One Finger

Do you remember how my German Shepherd, Isis, couldn't find me in my body and howled in the night? At first I was devastated, then I became irritated. A pair of mallard ducks flew into the backyard and decided my unkempt swimming pool was a little lake. Strangely they lay their eggs near the glass wall of my room.

After some time the mallard eggs in the nest beside my french doors were finally hatched, helped by the warmth of Isis' body as she spent each night sleeping with her body pressed against the doors. The ducklings concluded that this monster German Shepherd was their mother and followed her in a line all over the yard. The mallard parents didn't seem to mind, and they all got on peaceably. One day Isis was encouraged to bring the ducklings into the library to greet my body. The little ducklings huddled up against the bed and hushed their incessant low quackings. The Madonna of Fatima glowed. Sun bouncing off the water in the pool wove a web of golden light on the wall over my head, crowning me before these small creatures of the earth. Isis for once did not whine and beg to get out. Nor did she sniff at my body. She lay quietly on the floor and closed her eyes, accepting my disembodied being at last. Since this episode she has lost her pitiful harassed look and has regained her old dignity. It is a great triumph for me. I have finally gotten my mental being through to the natural world without my lack of a body getting in between. The little ducklings became ducks and flew away. Isis remained by my bed, at last my true constant companion.

Pat and Bill came in and saw Isis lying by my bed. Pat said with a rush of excitement as he watched Isis becoming more comfortable with my body. "This dog knows something that we don't."

Isis was right. I had been trying to embody my mind. My useless physical therapy was based on a physical approach to body. The health profession seemed to accept that mind had nothing to do with making body work.

How about using mind to make bodywork just for my mind? I had one simple practical goal. My mind needed one finger to push the keys on a normal computer. I had been gathering all my mental energy and concentration on moving one finger. So far the finger had not moved. Somehow Isis knew what I was trying to do and believed I could do it. She believed! Maybe with Pat and Bill here expecting something, I could finally break through. My head was propped up on a pillow and I could see my hand. I concentrated again, using everyone's mental energy.

I found myself looking at my finger – not my hand – the first finger. I was looking at my finger! I couldn't feel my body so I hadn't looked at it. Like Isis I saw this body attached to me as not being mine. Now I was seeing it as being my finger. I saw the curving length of my finger, the scaly skin, the ligaments, the loose, unused flesh. My finger.

It moved! My index finger moved up and down. By God, I did it!

"That's a miracle," Pat cries, "and it has all happened since you've come back to us."

Bill said, "You've been holding out on us, James. Tell us what is happening."

My screen flashes, *My finger moved this morning because my mind needs it to push computer keys. That's it. That's all. Don't expect my body to come back to life. I can't feel my finger. Just let whatever is going to happen, happen. I'm not pushing for more bodily life in general – only what I need. All I need is one finger.*

I was soon ensconced behind a normal computer with a keyboard. With a plastic extension attached to my finger, I am soon able to touch the letters and print my messages with my own finger. Just one finger. That's all.

Some weeks later Rachel Skouras from the hospital came by, "Congratulations, James. I've heard the good news. Nothing medically has changed, so obviously this physical improvement of yours has a mental vector. The news has been spreading in the hospital that what was considered impossible a short while ago is now possible. People who would have been given up as hopeless cases last year are showing unusual signs of improvement this year. The medication isn't different in the sense that there have been no breakthroughs. I believe it is simply that the mental atmosphere has changed since you have pointed the way. Some doctors have quietly accepted the power of informed patient participation. They are empowering patients and themselves."

Pat came in after Rachel left and regarded me somberly, "Is this really you or is it an imitation of the world's idea of you?"

Come on, Pat. This is wonderful news. Everyone is so excited now. Things will settle down.

Pat walks to the window, "I'm trying to be glad, God knows. I've been saying goodbye to the dear ghost I have come to love and getting ready to greet the old friend I loved in the flesh. But I must confess that I'm afraid. It's inevitable that as you become more involved with your body that you will misuse your mental power."

I typed, *But you haven't been around in some time, Pat. You don't know what has been going on. These people coming to see me — individual intimacy — individual growing — growing from inside out. More people are being affected in more ways and in more different places.*

Now listen to me very carefully. My body is going to be activated only as much as it is useful to me to do what I conceive I am here to do — and no more. I am no longer interested in my body only as body. Things are more complicated and wonderful than you have imagined. Come and join the crowd that comes around now. Exciting things are happening even though they may not be just as you had expected. Come on now.

Various organizations began asking for my input and participation, one of these was the Isthmus Institute, which is dedicated to exploring the convergence of science and the spirit. It brought speakers from around the world, including Noble laureates, to Dallas for meetings. Now, in a burst of faith in the spirit, the Isthmus Board of Trustees chose me to be president. How could a man without a body effectively preside over this internationally famous Institute? My message is essentially personal. Isthmus is involved with large meetings. It seems that the purpose of my survival is to leave a personal mes-

sage. However, the main purpose of Isthmus is to get the right mix of great thinkers from around the world. Maybe the unrealized purpose of Isthmus is to get individual great thinkers intimately involved with other great thinkers. The power generated by that intimacy may influence the audience more than any words they may speak. I could do that. Also I could communicate through email on my computer to talk to people all over the world. I will accept the presidency.

My Mental Universe

I'm free of my body now and being free of it makes it possible for me to use it for life-intentions. I'm not going to fight for bodily life so needlessly that I will fall into a terrible depression as I did before. Self as a mental entity beyond the body may become an intention directed toward "god." My visit to the wild universe seemingly burned away my former body images and I am left free to be aware of my compassionate self and my body and to know the difference.

Think about it. The body makes such preposterous demands upon the universe. If it is not kept within 10 degrees of its arbitrary temperature, it refuses to live. It must be constantly fueled and cleaned. It must have oxygen and water pumped into it. It becomes sick and tired. It pulls you down. But there will be a time soon when mind will be able to take flight and love its body at the same time.

At the moment most people react with horror to the possibility of a mind free of a body, but such a possibility does not limit us. It is no more horrible to have a mind with little body than to have a body with little mind. Having both possibilities in our future is better than only having one. As we pass through life we can be glad that as our bodies diminish, it is possible for our minds to expand.

Would we want to deny this mental possibility to others because we don't want it for ourselves? Body and mind each have their own values, and as we live, our lives are composed of both in varying degrees. The body's life is precious. Mental life is also precious. They are both precious absolutely. They are both beyond comparison with anything else.

I can only communicate with a particular person, in a particular time and place. In fact I can only communicate with a particular mind generating and being generated by a particular brain – or in some cases a particular fragment of a brain. Mind is the only real human diversity. Gender, black or yellow or brown skin only show how unimportant such surface diversity is. I seek the real mental person.

There is a final end to the body, but that is our own private end of mortality, not necessarily the end of personal mind. What we finally make of our minds is what is born from our bodies. With our bodies we begin. Our minds may never end.

Freud considered himself to have been an adventurer of the mind. Jung, my patron, thought of his work as an adventure to strange and exotic mindscapes. We think of these two men as the great figures of human science. They changed the way the world thinks. Yet adventurers into the dimension of mind, free of body, may change the world far more than they.

The first steps will be mapping the distinctions between mental patterns which depend on the body and mental patterns which exist independently of the body. Examples of body thoughts are all the ways we sense physical things – sight, sound, smell, and touch. An emotional state such as love, however, both is physical and mental. The point is knowing the difference for each and everyone of us. It would have been thought unlikely, but I have discovered that love survives the absence of the body and is only further enhanced. The mental being of compassionate conscious soul is the next place for humankind to evolve.

We are on the threshold of directly experiencing this mental universe. It is my feeling that if enough people have not reached this gateway to mental life soon, then it will be too late for our kind.

Conservation and capitalism become the same thing. Conservation becomes dictatorship. It's the only way to make people do what is best for the planet. Capitalism becomes dictatorship. It's the only way to control the complex global economy. Democracy becomes dictatorship. The role of government becomes too complex. The best people with the best programs do more evil than the worst people. Individual differences becomes the same. Everything becomes the same. This is a description of Death.

It makes a good deal of sense to consider that the world could indeed self-destruct. I don't mean self-destruct through war or ecological catastrophe, but simply because of a lack of trust in one another's intentions. It would be a mean, whining end to a species that has touched the heavens. Whatever pilgrimage of soul it will take to save humankind will begin on Earth and end in the universe of rushing mental forces.

Be in the world, not of it. You can be on the way to discover the release that comes from knowing that you cannot control the wild universe, but you can be redeemed by your truly unique compassionate intentions – no matter what happens to you.

But remember, making a compassionate intention may be a terrible mistake if the compassion is a mistake. Following rules will not save us. We personally are responsible for our salvation.

Patton Howell   James Hall

VIII

Redeemed

Redemption

This is Patton writing the last chapter. It has been ten years now since James' stroke had left him without body sensations. Tonight was a big night for him. I met Susy and James at the Southwestern Health Science Center on the outskirts of Dallas where James was once a professor. The Center was a magic place. It embraced three hospitals, one of the great medical schools, an internationally famous research center with a number of Nobel Laureates on its staff. On overhead tramways people were whisked from one cluster of glass towers to another.

It was dark when I pulled up at the entrance guard house and explained we would have to deposit James there by the auditorium. I would park the van and come back to get him and Susy. When I returned Susy pushed him across a bridge into the curving shadowy vastness of the auditorium lobby. Eager hands took him into the auditorium.

Susy stayed in the lobby. Suddenly there was nothing to do — everything was well organized and so many people dedicated to James. The trouble is they didn't seem to realize that just getting James here is more trouble than organizing this event.

This is the fall conference of the Isthmus Institute and James is now its president. This meeting will last three days and will be a revisioning of the place of psychology in the life of the spirit. With his computer James has written and explained and persuaded, Nobel laureates, heads of churches, and distinguished scholars from over the world who have come at his call. How can a paralyzed man with only one finger run a huge international organization? Easy. Delegate. The only problem so far is that the staff is always exhausted. The boss never sleeps.

I had gone in to confer with James. The auditorium is a curving half circle of seats dropping down amphitheater-style to a stage dominated by a twelve foot screen. Everything is plush and gleamingly automated.

The bright lights from the auditorium spill through an open door into the dimly lit lobby along with the buzz of excitement and the sound of applause. I came through the door looking for Susy and saw her standing in the shadowed lobby. I strode over to her and put an arm around her shoulders, "Susy, things are getting started. You must come in now. You will be missed."

Susy turned her face up to me. "I think I had better straighten you out, Pat. James is teaching others a new way of being in the world, a renewal of themselves, a redemption, but as important he is teaching these things to himself. He seeks redemption for himself and his life. You and Bill are so busy listening to his words, you can't hear how he has changed himself since he came back – changed the very roots of his being. I have been changing my being as well. You haven't heard me changing in myself any more than you have James."

She goes on, "My fantasy was that one day James would realize his selfishness, his betrayals, his self-centered life, and he would come to me and confess and humbly ask my forgiveness. He hasn't done that, and he won't. I'm glad. What has happened is better. As soon as he came back I realized that the self-centeredness was gone. He is centered beyond himself and beyond me. He is struggling with how to do that in this world. But the big thing for me was that I was freed from the suffocation of being dominated by him. Now he didn't expect or assume anything from me."

Suddenly, Susy had all my attention.

She shot a sharp glance at me. "You haven't even noticed, have you? I've helped him when it was convenient, but if I'm too tired or the house needs attention or if I feel the need just to go out, I do. If he needs attention, I'm not necessarily available. You haven't even noticed. It isn't that he's given me anything. I have the freedom to take what I need. I'm free to move out of his structure, and I'm free to move back in. For the first time, maybe, in my life I'm free to love him, and I do love him. I want the best for him. He is a man with an important vision."

I was stunned. How could I have been so insensitive? "I know the program tonight, and I know what James' computer will say. He will portray you as the one true thing in his life, that you have saved him. Everything that happens tonight he will attribute to your influence. I didn't understand this at first, but I do now. He brings to you the love of the universe."

I noticed for the first time that Susy had acquired an inner peace. The lines of her face had smoothed out. Her body had stilled, her eyes were steady on my face. She seemed to know her place in the universe far beyond what I had achieved.

She turned to me. "I don't like the noise and excitement. I got him here. I'm happy for him and for me. I want to live here in the shadow. It has its own compassion."

Susy, herself, seemed in the shadow to be glowing with a heavenly radiance. She was the one out of all the people here who was actually being redeemed.

Susy and I remained in the quiet lobby. The lights and excitement in the auditorium went on.

Locked In To Life

Appendix

James' Universe

Vision #1: The Beginning

The universe has a beginning. There are seven levels. The universe began as a singularity. But I discovered that the beauty of a singularity of thought was a Great Thought – rather than a Big Bang. The beauty of a time that was always becoming into an expanding future. The past was always becoming, and "now" was its becomingness.

Complex relationships of thought best describe what occurred in the first split second of the universe. Some mathematical equations describe this moment using only tangible, physical relationships. However, much of mathematics is "pure" in the sense that it is immaterial. It often does not describe real physical relationships. Pure mathematics best describes what was intangibly present at the split second after the beginning – intangible thought.

Vision #2: A Great Thought

Everything that happened at the beginning of the universe is in reality still with us. Nothing more can be added or subtracted from the universe. Everything that exists now had to be there at the start. That doesn't seem possible physically, but it is possible mentally. The beginning was a Great Thought moving out, the whorls of itself caused by its expansion coalescing into stars but always connected by its thought. The universe has been bathed in elemental thought since the beginning. James Jeans, an astronomer and physicist, agrees with me. He said that, the universe reminded him of a great thought more than a great machine. Thus in the becomingness of the beginning – pure immaterial mathematics became overlaid with the first physical "matter."

Vision #3: Immortal Elemental Matter

When physicists use a grate with several slots, nuclear particles will often go through the slot physicists expect them to – as though reacting to the physicists thoughts. Sometimes they are immaterial waves, and sometimes they are particles, flickering between the energy, thought and of the energy of matter. Quantum particles flicker between mind and matter, and to the flickering thought becomes veils of rushing colors. My vision of color is red, yellow, green, blue, and purple. The beginning veils are red.

What is a black hole? Imagine running the universe backwards. Elementary particles can partly escape from a black hole that allows no material to escape. Going backward primal mental energy escapes. The thought aspect of elemental particles is to escape. Black holes deteriorate and return energy to the universe. This energy is mental flickering back and forth between elemental thought and elemental matter.

Vision #4: The Relationships of Molecular Matter

As time progresses, these elemental particles are overlaid by elemental relationships. They become randomly connected molecules rather than individual elemental particles. Time is beginning to show a direction. These relationships are not immortal. Individually they break down and then reform at random.

Who pushes whom around. The elemental particles get pushed around the most by the patterns of thought – or relationships – which evolved as the molecules of chemistry. Then the molecules get pushed around by the cells which have organized their relationships into a body. Even brain cells do not have much say about the direction of their fire. Those orders come from a higher command of ideas.

Vision # 5: Molecular Matter

Thought pervades the life-like relationships of molecular mat-ter – in red-streaked yellow. The beauty of biological life. Thought-structural molecules join together and lead to organic matter and cells. Life is not a new creation. It is a further devel-opment of the immaterial beginning. In the first split second of creation The Great Thought began to clothe its extension in mat-ter. For example, the DNA code of every cell has been a message about relationships. The message has been written down on amino acids. We think of the transmission of life as a physical sex-ual passing on of genes. But the genes are merely the material message of an immaterial thought. Life is made of patterns of thought written on molecules of DNA.

Vision #6: Human Beings

We encounter the beauty of human beings. Since the beginning Great Thought the rate of change of the mental universe has accelerated exponentially. Human thought has used matter as a mirror to see its own message. In the thousands of years since the beginning, as personal human lives have been developing, physical matter has become a page upon which to write thoughts, a mirror in which to see ourselves. "I" the essential human being, is thought.

Vision #7: A Return to the Beginning of the Universe

Human beings finds themselves on the threshold of a communion with the beginning Great Thought. The self connects in a feedback loop to the beginning of the universe. It is mental, not physical. This is the moment when I communicated with that mental presence out in the wild rush of universal thought. It is where I find my ultimate sense of peace and serenity. This is when I reached my new understanding of life and my task of redemption.

Locked In To Life

The Brain

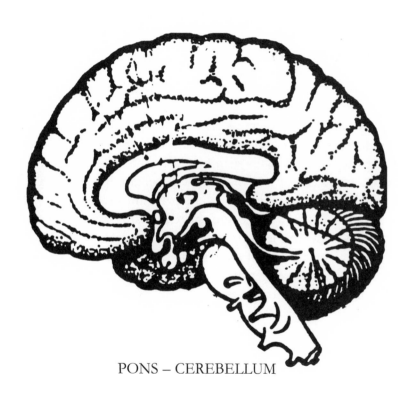

PONS – CEREBELLUM

The Locked-in Syndrome

The membrane enclosing the brain tissue is like a plastic baggie. We're looking at the cortex. Here is the left hemisphere and its twin right hemisphere. One of these hemispheres – half of the cortex – could be missing and there would be little difference in the person's life. What we call thinking uses a very small part of the brain.

We can expose the pons area underneath the cortex by using this stainless steel shoehorn. You see, we work under and around the cortex and lift it up slightly and to the side. There is a gap between the cortex and the pons-cerebellum. The pons is not a unified structure like the cortex. Its parts are strewn about before us. These configurations are switch boards mediating neural impulses between the body and suitable areas of the cortex.

Below this mid-brain there is the medulla oblongata; our first brain. It is a thickening of the spinal column, the spinal nerve. This first brain controls basic body functions like breathing. We have three brains, each having evolved on top of the other. Evolution does not replace, it simply adds on. Our next evolution of the brain, the mid-brain, was added on top of the medulla and included the pons-cerebellum. The cortex, added on top of the other two brains was the final and modern addition to the brain.

In the Locked-in Syndrome the mid-brain is destroyed, but the lower brain below the mid-brain is not seriously affected. This allows the body to continue functioning even though the more complex cortex has been cut off from communication with it. The body moreover is able to supply blood to the cortex to keep it alive.

The symptoms that signify Locked-in Syndrome are as follows:

1) The body is paralyzed from the eyes down. It is as though one were a quadriplegic, but also unable to talk.

2) One's eyes are not paralyzed since they are connected to the remaining cells of the cortex, but there is initially little control of horizontal movement.

3) There is also facial paralysis.

Brain Dead

There are those who have lived a life of physical action whose minds become immobilized if their bodies are immobilized. Others have lived in a separate mental dimension, and their minds do not seem to be affected by physical immobility. These people, fine-tuned their minds when they had a body, so if their body is lost, their thoughts do not depend on their own particular brain any more than a fine piano player must depend on a particular piano.

The idea of the expression "brain-dead" referring to mental functions is no longer tenable. There are other alternatives. Brain-dead is an unfortunate and cruel metaphor. There is not a simple relationship between mind and brain. That relationship varies enormously. How many brain cells are dead? How few brain cells does it take to think. Is there a continuum of life which varies from an extreme state in which the mind gladly dies along with the body to extreme cases at the other end of the continuum like James in which mind even becomes enhanced without body? How much of life exists as subconscious. We can drive a car with nothing but subconscious thinking stimulus bound to traffic, stop signs and so on, hardly conscious of what we are doing. But James has no subconscious thinking because he has no body. The subconscious can only exist in terms of body behavior such as driving a car.

Mind Research

James feels he has eliminated all of his brain except the upper regions of his cortex as being necessary for his thinking self. Japanese neurologists have used cerebral blood flow measures by single photon emission tomography to study persistent vegetative states including Locked-in Syndrome. They were able to correlate awareness only with frontal lobe function. Their evidence was that alteration of cerebral blood flow occurred only in the frontal region. It appears that the purely conscious mind may use only cells in the upper and front regions of the cortex.

The question comes down first to what support system those particular brain cells need. James' experience has shown that the only necessity is a stable blood supply. Such a support system capable of indefinitely extended operation is certainly a possibility in the future. The technology required exists now. It would be only a matter of putting it together.

Mind

James' mind is all around us. It permeates us. Nevertheless James has been dependent on material tools to voice his immaterial thoughts. But don't we all do the same thing? When did you last have your dishwasher serviced, your car, your telephone, your TV, your heart or lungs – or as you get older your prostate? We are increasingly surrounded by tools that service our minds – even replace our bodies in the service of our minds. The increased services that James' mind requires are negligible compared to the support all of us already depend on. In fact, compared to the costs of an active body's life, the support of a disembodied mind like James' is negligible. This is just one aspect of how alien his being is, even to us. He doesn't need all the life support we take for granted.

Take for example clothes, food. James has two robes to clothe his body. But from his point of view he has no body. He doesn't care about his body. He gets some basic liquid foods poured into his intestines. But he doesn't care. He is not involved in body's life. He is like a hermit.

The ancient Egyptians believed that you could exchange body parts without changing the core personality. A stone scarab was routinely substituted for the heart in the mummification process. We have a similar practice in the form of organ donors in our own day. But does this alienate us from our bodies? We are in a position now to replace nearly all of the organs of the body. A person can have exchanged by transplant his or her most important body organs – heart, lungs, liver and kidneys – even bones and muscles – and yet they experience no change in mental being, in mind, soul, spirit or self. The consciousness of the person receiving the organ is not changed. Of course, we do not yet have anything as complicated as a brain transplant. But James' personal experience right now indicates that a brain transplant might turn out the same way.

What if we were able to transplant someone else's pontine mid-brain, to the pontine area where James experienced his stroke? There is no evidence to indicate that the self we would encounter after the operation would not be James' own self. In other words, the pontine mid-brain is not necessary for James' mental self, nor is it necessary for the survival of the body. The medulla oblongata, the primitive brain, is necessary to the survival of the body, but has little influence on the mind.

What is left is James' partially damaged cortex. This is his third and most evolutionarily advanced brain. The only physical location left for his thinking is the cortex. However, there is no physiological map which purports to locate one's mental being over the entire cortex. Perhaps James' mental self is attributable to only a part of the cortex.

Solid research evidence that the comparatively few cells used in mental intentions are located in a small area of the brain called the Supplemental Motor Area. It is located right at the top of your head. There is reason to believe that these cells act more as transmitters and transformers of mental intentions whose genesis lie outside the brain rather than as the creators of such intentions.

As the mother's womb is for the baby, perhaps one's body is a womb for the mind. Perhaps at some point we don't need our bodies anymore just as the baby doesn't need the womb. What functions does the body perform after we've matured? What does it do for us? Every bodily physical function – lifting, moving, pulling, kicking – can be performed better by a machine. Building a bionic body makes no sense. A bionic mind does – a limited number of brain cells supporting a living personal mind could be maintained with available electronic machinery.

Pure Consciousness

In pure consciousness there is no unconscious thinking. How could God, for instance, have unconscious thinking? God would be pure consciousness. Pure consciousness engulfs the subconscious. Self is at last pure and whole. All the psychological terms we use to describe the self become psychobabble. They are really only about the body's self. Mind without body is such an alien existence that it has been very hard for us to even contemplate.

In spite of the scientific culture of the last few hundred years, the perdurable instinct of people remains that each of us has an existence beyond our bodies. We still believe that there is something immaterial about who we are, something about our selves that could extend beyond the dissolution of the body. The soul for which mankind has been yearning over the millennia has finally become accessible. James has brought back the human soul to live in harmony with the body and mature out of it. Jung would be pleased. One of Jung's paintings depicts this occurrence, the soul becoming accessible in life as it is lived – not as a mystical belief, but as a comfortable reality.

Spirit is not attained by following rules but by following personal guides like James who have lived spiritual lives themselves. It is not necessary to suffer from a Locked-in Syndrome, nor is it necessary to go so far as sensory deprivation.

James has actually recovered the reality of soul from the mysticism of religion. Soul can live in harmony with the body in the every day life of the scientific age. Soul can now be the subject of scientific research. It is clear and undeniable that while brain cells may act as valves and conduits for the expression of thought, they are not consciousness itself. Consciousness is simply the fundamental reality of the universe. Consciousness is everywhere. It may exist in primitive forms such as gravity, for example. Gravity exists everywhere. One may say that gravity is so unthinkably powerful that it holds the entire universe together. Yet gravity is immaterial. It has no body. It is not made of matter.

How little one thinks of the possibility of living as pure consciousness of soul at the beginning of this odyssey. James had been the quintessential sensualist, steeped in all the lusts of flesh. After his accident he would have lost all sense of his body. His thinking would have unravelled into the universe if he had not had, in addition to a strong body, a strong highly disciplined mind. He fought and struggled; he threatened heaven and earth for his soul. His legacy for all of us is that possibility.

Epistemological Question

The experience of a human self is provided in the social context of each individual, even before birth, bringing that individual into the stream of an on-going message of who she is and what she is doing here.

In the modern period, we have witnessed personal self transcending biological evolution. This personal development of the individual makes possible a self with a fluid edge. First humans living in an alien world depended for survival on passing on rituals of dance, music and poetry. As the natural world became dominated by human-made civilizations, changes in self appeared.

There was at that time a conflict between the static atomic philosophy of Democritus and the panta rhei (everything flows) view of Heraclitus. Heraclitus, known as the Dark Philosopher, was from a rich Ephesian family. He believed that self was change. All things were becoming. Democritus, on the other hand, known as the Laughing Philosopher, was from Thrace and was poor. His method was to reduce change to an irreducible static construct which he called an "atom." Democritus won. Human science has since clung tightly to the idea of a world composed of static objective reducible structures.

Two epistemological questions. First: How is it possible for the self to change its essential quality of being? Second: How can we know if the self has changed its essential quality of being?

Epistemological questions have traditionally been contained within systems of static objective reducible systems. This method culminated in Isaac Newton's calculus. Calculus attempts to objectify continuous change by allowing small static measures to represent the illusion of movement. But this method cannot take into account discontinuous changes such as a change in the self's essential quality of being. The Darwinian theory of small continuous changes determined by natural selection is being replaced by theories of saltational discontinuity in evolution and others. Human science has a qualitative answer. The continuity of self has been constantly changing throughout mental evolution. The accumulation of subjective change in a static rational society produces discontinuous change of self.

The second question, how could we know if a discontinuous change in self had occurred, can be referred to current changes in mathematical theory. This thinking is returning to the "panta rhei" (reality is flow) philosophy of Heraclitus in theories which appeal to non-linear, multi-dimensional models of thought. An example is chaos theory which can treat an essence of self as a "strange attractor," whose repeated subjective interactions are accompanied by unpredictable discontinuous change.

This brings up the third epistemological question, if we do discover people whose selves have changed catastrophically, how will we be able to nurture them and help them develop? That is the challenge which the authors of this book are attempting to meet.

Ancient Meter

Words changed. The story changed. But ritual rhythms remained, and the subtle energies evoked by the rhythms remained. These were powers to see into one's own self. Only humankind had been given this ability. But there was no gene for this gift. It could only be reproduced in each generation through passing on rhythmic rituals of dance, music, drama, poetry.

You absorbed the surviving true selves of people, which were passed on to you over tens of thousands of years. You became the physical hands of those without bodies. They wait to live in you. Lacking bodies now, they feel for you and care for you still. They are unselfish precisely because they have no bodies.

Take their feeling hands into your feeling hands in a connection of warm, intimate touching.

When you begin to perceive yourself as inner shapes, what do you do with them? They don't fit together in a linear sequence on a two dimensional page like this. They transcend time and space. Our most advanced researchers are now seeking meanings in non-linear multi-dimensional computational shapes in chaos theory, fuzzy logic and especially in complexity theory.

Ascribing shapes to subtle energies seems fanciful, but it can be as real as the shape of your body and the shapes you can see and feel around you. Sometimes your feelings are as misty and amorphous as clouds and blow past without your noticing. But also you have an ability to find precise inner shapes in your misty feelings. You can live with your inner self as well as you can live in the objective world. You can enrich your life by knowing your self in all its precise colors and dimensions.

Think of a time, for instance, when you had a problem but were not thinking about it rationally. Your mind was a blank. Upon that blank of mind feeling tones, patterns and connections began to take shape. Your problem was solved by multi-dimensional shapes of feelings. Afterwards you used linear language to explain what had happened and actually came to believe that you had solved the problem through rational thinking.

The only quality necessary to the power of your inner self is wonder. Fortunately all human beings have this quality. It is what distinguishes us from the other animals. It is why we are destined for the stars. Rational thought is useful, but it has not created our true selves. Wonder has made us human, and wonder is a feeling. If it did not come first, rational objectivity would have no purpose.

Shamanistic myths through the ages tell of the two faces each person has. One face is physical and is presented to the world. The other face is the ethereal face of power and one spends one's life seeking to meet this finally true self.

A living self can become intimate and warm. It can be created from the shapes of the pure rush of living selves. Our whole and true selves can become feeling guides we can always trust.

You can trust your self; then you exist no matter what happens to you. You are part of it all. No matter what you do or think, you will exist absolutely.

People are always defending themselves. If they knew that they existed absolutely in their own inner selves, they would need no defense.

Changing Minds

There is a foreseeable future of minds evolving beyond bodies. Is it our future? One thing seems clear – behaviorism, which does not infer a subjective state but relies only on what behavior can be observed, seems unable to deal with the complexity of James' mental condition. He has shown little externally observable behavior yet he possesses a rich mental life.

There seems no way out of relying on subjective reports such as this case history of James Hall contaminated as it must be by prior assumptions and experiences. But the great philosopher of the nineties, Michael Polanyi, has pointed out that if we cannot escape the habit of relying on observers then let us at least rely on good observers who are trained to report their experiences as objectively as possible. In that regard James has been in a unique position since all of his training and practice has been in sorting out mental patterns.

The purpose of a stable body-image is largely practical – to be aware of the body's disposition in space, to keep from bumping into other things. If you cannot move the body, if it is merely a machine to pump blood to the brain, what difference does its image make There is no necessity for the usual moment-to-moment awareness of the body's position in space. Nevertheless, James tried to maintain a body-image in his mind even though he was disembodied. This led him into a paroxysm of selfishness which became depression and finally led to his desperate and suicidal exploration into the rushing mental universe.

The fact that the one-to-one correspondence between body and body-image are not the same is shown by the phenomena of phantom limbs. When a limb is amputated, after about a year and a half, (it takes that long) there are frequently "phantom" sensations that seem to come from the missing limb as if it still existed. The usual explanation is that the severed nerves continue to send impulses which are interpreted as if they came from the original terminus of the nerves in the missing limb. Nerves are even surgically sectioned in some cases in an attempt to remove the phantom sensations. The trouble is that nerves and nerve tracts in the spinal cord can be severed right up to the brain itself without altering the phantom sensations. The body-image (the "phantom") is apparently more persistent than the actual body itself!

The psychology of pure disembodied consciousness is a new untouched realm of mental experience. It's research methodologies are simple and direct as were those in the great days of the physical sciences. As Rollo May said about James, "Mind is finally cleansed of the corruptions of body and brain. Mind is finally available for direct study. The absurd attempts to study mind by studying something entirely different – behavior – can be laid to rest. Because it has been too difficult to study the mind, we have studied behavior instead and had the temerity to call it psychology."

The Future

If there have been people among us with newly evolved kinds of minds, we have been unaware of them because we have little language to inquire into a mind changing its essential quality of being.

Some people today can include all experience within their minds. If their bodies were made alien in a holocaust their minds would still be human. These new people are comfortable living with ambiguity. They can proceed with and believe in projects which have no end or beginning and which may involve simultaneous contradictions. They can break rules and at the same time use those rules as preconditions for their work.

They have available technological tools which give them unlimited access to information and knowledge. And they are able to be very good simultaneously in different disciplines.

New minds transcend interior boundaries and social walls of wealth, education, sex, race, profession, religion and class – not by making everyone the same, but by having more interior room for each other in all their maddening differences. These new minds have developed simultaneous multiple loyalties. They can be loyal to various aspects of their countries and to various aspects of the ecology of the world, but they are indifferent to ideologies.

There are people living today who can cherish and preserve diversity but transcend the walls built by others to defend those diversities against change.

Their environmental concerns are natural and personal rather than political. They are free of cultural morals, yet they have fidelity for themselves and care for others. They have no ego center, yet everything falls inward. They have selves with fluid edges.

Religions have envisioned an unchangeable God-made precious vessel to contain and preserve the self and to sail away with it beyond our horizons, unchanged after death. Psychology has accepted the concept of a Freudian-inspired static self of irreducible parts – as though there were a super-ego, ego, id, to give static structure to the self and preserve it.

Today people have gone beyond the static structures of psychology. They are ready to experience James' wild universe.

Locked In To Life

A Personal Note

We, Susy, James, Bill, Patton hope that the readers of our story have found inspiration to understand the beauty of mind without body. James' experience shows how a stroke can be an opportunity to be reborn into a better life. Our story is really a work constantly in progress, but this seemed a likely place to interrupt it and to publish this book. We are all in this human exploration together. Perhaps we can keep in touch.

Please feel free to write to Patton Howell or James Hall.

Patton Howell and/or James Hall
c/o Tea Road Press
Please check the www.tearoadpress.com web site for address.

Resources

Please note that all information is as accurate as possible at the time of publication. We have listed both the American Stroke Association and the National Stroke Association in our resources. These two organizations frequently work together to advocate on issues affecting those with stroke.

Stroke Information

Keeping in mind that there is never one cause for a particular stroke, here are some conditions for stroke occurrence. The following information should be considered as general and any concerns you have should be addressed by your physician.

1.   High blood pressure: Average blood pressure is 130/85. A person with a blood pressure of 160/95 is four times more likely to have a stroke than a person with average blood pressure. Recent investigations show that reducing the resting pressure, say from 85 to 80 could reduce stroke by forty percent.

2.   Irregular heart rhythms: These can allow clots to collect in the heart. From the heart, the clots can be carried to the brain and cause a stroke. About one stroke in four is caused by heart irregularities. Thinning your blood by taking a drug such as Coumadin may cut the likelihood of a stroke from irregular heart beating by fifty percent.

3.   High Cholesterol: Cholesterol can build up deposits on the inside of arteries. Such build-ups can contribute to blocking blood supply to brain cells. Staying below the 200 level of cholesterol is desirable to help present strokes. Controlling fat consumed, and especially the saturated fat, in ones diet is the way to hold down the cholesterol level.

4.   Smoking: Stroke risk for people who smoke sixty cigarettes a day is four times greater than those who smoke less than ten cigarettes per day. At least in terms of strokes, switching to cigars or pipes does not lower the risk.

5.   Alcohol: People who have more than two drinks per day double their risk of having a stroke.

Know the Warning Signs of Stroke

One or more of the following signs in another person or yourself should prompt immediate medical attention for stroke treatment.

1. Sudden numbness or weakness of the face, arm or leg, especially on one side of the body
2. Sudden confusion, trouble speaking or understanding
3. Sudden trouble seeing in one or both eyes
4. Sudden trouble walking, dizziness, loss of balance or coordination
5. Sudden, severe headache with no known cause

Not all of these signs occur with every stroke. Sometimes they go away and return. If some occur, get help fast. If you notice one or more of these signs in another person, don't wait. Call 9-1-1 and get them to a hospital right away.

What is a TIA (transient ischemic attack)?

A TIA is a "mini-stroke" with the same signs as a stroke, only the signs last only a few minutes. About 10 percent of strokes are preceded by TIAs. However, of those who have had one or several TIAs, about 36 percent will later have a stroke TIAs are extremely important stroke warning signs. Don't ignore them. Call 911 or go to your emergency room immediately.

American Stroke Association

National Center
7272 Greenville Avenue
Dallas, Texas 75231

1-888-4-STROKE
or 1-888-478-7653
www.strokeassociation.org

The American Stroke Association is committed to reducing disability and death from stroke through research, education, fund raising and advocacy. A Division of the American Heart Association, the agency offers a wide array of programs, products and services, from patient education materials to current scientific statements and reports for healthcare professionals. Life after stroke, resources and access to support groups throughout the nation for survivors, caregivers, and healthcare professionals are available through the American Stroke Association's Stroke Family Support Network.

National Stroke Association

National Center
9707 E. Easter Lane
Englewood, Colorado 80112

Toll Free: 1-800-STROKES
Phone: 303-649-9299
www.stroke.org

The National Stroke Association provides national expertise and leadership for those at risk, suffering or recovering from this devastating condition. Began in 1984, the National Stroke Association is aggressively taking steps to reduce the incidence and impact of stroke. In communities across the country this association helps people understand the urgency for symptom recognition. We are teaching them how to respond and are partnering with professionals from a variety of disciplines to improve quality of care and patient outcomes.

American Heart Association

American Heart Association
National Center
7272 Greenville Avenue
Dallas,Texas 75231

1-800-AHA-USA-1
or 1-800-242-8721
www.americanheart.org

The American Heart Association is a non-profit organization where information on diet, exercise and heart healty habits can be found. The American Heart Association sponsors numerous public service programs and sources of information. There programs create public awareness which leads to increased visibility and education on issues relating to public health.

The National Aphasia Association

National Aphasia Association
29 John St., Suite 1103
New York, NY 10038

1-800-922-4622
www.aphasia.org

Aphasia is an inability to use or comprehend words, often associated with impairment resulting from a stroke. Further information regarding this condition can be found at the web site for the National Aphasisa Association.

Social Security

www.sssa.gov

The Social Security Nationwide Toll-Free Telephone Service number is 1-800-772-1213. Information on supplemental security income or disability benefits; free literature on retirement benefits, disability benefits, Medicare, and survivor benefits.

The Job Accommodation Network

http://www.jan.wvu.edu/
Job Accommodation Network
1-800-526-7234 (V/TTY)

The Job Accommodation Network (JAN) is a free consulting service that provides information about job accommodations, the Americans with Disabilities Act (ADA), and the employability of people with disabilities.

What does JAN do? JAN is the most comprehensive resource for job accommodations available. JAN consultants provide information on accommodation ideas for workers with disabilities, what products are available to accommodate individuals, and where these products can be purchased. JAN consultants also provide information on the ADA. Consultants provide this information by fax, e-mail, and postal mail.

Office of Disease Prevention and Health Promotion

U.S. Department of Health and Human Services
Office of Disease Prevention and Health Promotion
200 Independence Avenue SW, Room 738G
Washington, DC 20201
202.401.6295 (Voice)
202.205.9478 (Fax)

Works to strengthen the disease prevention and health promotion priorities of the Department of Health within the collaborative framework of the HHS agencies. Excellent source of extended information regarding health and support services.

Mended Hearts

7272 Greenville Avenue, Dallas
Texas 75231-4596
214.706.1442 (Voice)
214.706.5231 (Fax)
http://www.mendedhearts.org/purpose.html

Mended Hearts, Inc. is proud to be affiliated with the American Heart Association. Both organizations support each others goals and objectives and are committed to helping heart disease patients and families/caregivers.

We are an extended support group for heart patients, families and caregivers. Available to speak to heart disease patients about what they are going through. A network of people who have heart disease. Families or caregivers of heart patients, who are available to speak to your family members going through the same experience.

Available in 260 cities across the U.S. and in Sudbury, Ontario, Canada. Mended Hearts is a support organization composed of a special group of people: heart patients, spouses, health professionals and other interested persons. Mended Hearts is particularly interested in helping people deal with the emotional recovery from heart disease.

Patton Howell

Books by Patton Howell:

Embodied Mind

Fully Alive, Golden Pen Award

Novel Prize Conversations, Editor

Methods, Editor, PEN, Essay Award

Beyond Literacy, Editor, Benjamin Franklin Award

Napa Valley, Editor

Self Through Art and Science with Patton Howell

Stroke as Metamorphosis

The Terrorist Mind, PEN Award

War's End

Locked In To Life, with James Hall

James Hall

Books by James Hall:

Clinical Uses of Dreams: Jungian Interpretations and
  Enactments, reissued as Patterns of Dreaming

The Jungian Experience: Analysis and Individuation

Jung's Self Psychology: A Constuctivist Perspective

The Unconscious Christian: The Image of God in Dreams

Hypnosis: A Jungian Perspective

Clinical Hypnosis: Principles and Applications (2nd Edition)

Jungian Dream Interpretation: A Handbook of Theory and Practice

Self Through Art and Science with Patton Howell

The Book of the Self, edited with Polly Jung-Eisendrath

Locked In To Life, with Patton Howell

Locked In To Life

Index